ATKINS DIET COOKBOOK

The Easy Steps to Follow Guide to Understand Atkins Meal Plan

(Beginners Guide on Shedding Weight and Living Healthy)

Robert Decker

Published by Alex Howard

© **Robert Decker**

All Rights Reserved

Atkins Diet Cookbook: The Easy Steps to Follow Guide to Understand Atkins Meal Plan (Beginners Guide on Shedding Weight and Living Healthy)

ISBN 978-1-990169-66-3

All rights reserved. No part of this guide may be reproduced in any form without permission in writing from the publisher except in the case of brief quotations embodied in critical articles or reviews.

Legal & Disclaimer

The information contained in this book is not designed to replace or take the place of any form of medicine or professional medical advice. The information in this book has been provided for educational and entertainment purposes only.

The information contained in this book has been compiled from sources deemed reliable, and it is accurate to the best of the Author's knowledge; however, the Author cannot guarantee its accuracy and validity and cannot be held liable for any errors or omissions. Changes are periodically made to this book. You must consult your doctor or get professional medical advice before using any of the suggested remedies, techniques, or information in this book.

Table of contents

Part 1 1

Introduction 2

Atkins Desserts Recipes 84

Black Velvet Cupcakes 84

Caramelized Pear Custard 86

Cardamom Butter Cookies 88

Cherry Cobbler 90

Cherry Hazelnut Biscotti 92

Chocolate And Flan Layered Mini Cakes 93

Chocolate Donut Delight 95

Chocolate Ice Cream 97

Chocolate Mint Cheesecake Bars 98

Chocolate Mousse Mini Cheesecakes 100

Chocolate Mudslide 102

Chocolate Peanut Butter Haystacks 102

Chocolate Peppermint Cupcakes 103

Chocolate Walnut Cookies 105

Chocolate Yule Log 106

Chocolate-Cappuccino Mini Cupcakes 108

Chocolate-Coconut Haystacks 109

Chocolate-Cream Frosty 110

Chocolate-Ginger Cake 110

Chocolate-Mint Mousse Layer Cake 112

Chocolate-Peanut Whip 114

Chunky Mocha Ice Cream 114

Cinnamon Custard 116

Cinnamon-Almond Meringues 117

Classic Apple Tart 118

Classic Chocolate Cupcakes 119

Coconut Cookies 121

Coconut Lemon Ice Cream With Blackberry-Peach Compote .. 122

Coconut Macaroons 124

Coconut Panna Skullotta 125

Coconut Shortcakes With Berries And Cream 126

Coconut-Cashew Chocolate Truffles 127

Coconut-Lime Mousse 129

Coeur A La Creme 129

Coffee Eggnog 131

Cranberry Parfait 131

Cranberry-Raspberry Gelatin Dessert 132

Part 2 134

Introduction 135

Apricot-Glazed Roasted Asparagus (Low Fat) 136

Quick Low-Fat Mushrooms 137

Very Simple Oven Fried Chicken -- Low Fat 139

Crustless Spinach Quiche (Low Fat) 140

Low Fat Spinach And Artichoke Dip 141

Broccoli Cheese Soup - 20 Minute Fast And Low Fat 143

Lower Calorie Chicken Piccata 144

Low Cal Dill Sauce For Poached Fish 145

Low Carb Kfc Coleslaw 146

Chocolate Pudding, Low Fat 147

Low Fat Chili Made With Fat-Free Ground Turkey, 210 Calories Per 149

Low-Fat Burgundy Beef & Vegetable Stew 151

Cauliflower Salad Made Like Potato Salad (Low Carb) 152

Hash Browns (Patties - Low Sodium) Homemade 153

Chilled Strawberry Romance: The Soup (Low Fat) 154

Low-Fat, Low-Calorie, Jalapeno Cornbread 155

Easiest Low Fat French Fries 158

Crustless Tomato And Basil Quiche (Low Carb) 159

Fish Veronique (Low Fat, Diabetic Friendly) 160

Low Carb Pizza - Zucchini "Crust" 162

Low-Fat Scalloped Potatoes 163

Chewy Lower Fat Brownies 164

Low Country Zucchini And Yellow Squash 166

Easy Low-Fat Creamy Dill Salmon 167

Low-Fat Gravy 168

Low-Fat Chicken With Caramelized Onions 169

Chewy Lower Fat Brownies 171

Low Country Zucchini And Yellow Squash 172

Easy Low-Fat Creamy Dill Salmon..173

Low-Fat Gravy...174

Low-Fat Chicken With Caramelized Onions 175

Low-Fat Carnitas 176

Low-Carb Crab Cakes 178

Low Carb Lasagna 179

Low Cal Sole..181

Low Fat Sweet Apple 182

Apple Pie Parfait- Big On Taste, Not Calories! 183

Simple Sweet Potato Or Pumpkin Muffins (Low Calorie).........184

Jalapeno Rice- Low Fat...185

Part 1

Introduction

This book sheds light on why the Atkins diet is an unhealthy and deadly diet and also elucidates how making poor dietary choices will comprise your overall health. Moreover, appetizing healthy food recipes for improving your health which are easy to prepare are delineated in this book. Furthermore, how to substantially reduce risks for deadly chronic diseases by embracing a heart healthy, anticancer, nutrient dense, alkaline, antioxidant rich, anti-inflammatory raw fruitarian diet is expounded upon in this book. The Atkins diet is often erroneously touted as a healthy diet even though it is fraught with dietary issues that encompass rendering the consumption of ample unhealthy foods permissible, such as animal products and dairy products. Much to the chagrin of dieters, an exorbitant amount of non-alkaline, carcinogenic, acidic, pathogenic, cholesterol laced, endocrine distributive, inflammatory, and chronic disease promoting that are rendered permissible under the Atkins diet. The Atkins diet is unequivocally an unhealthy, deadly, and disease promoting diet for a myriad of reasons. The Atkins diet renders the consumption of ample foods that profusely ravage the DNA, shorten the telomeres, unravel the chromosomes, comprise all facets of your health, elicit chronic diseases, draw forth severe inflammation, and that decrease your longevity rate permissible. In other words, nothing salubrious can ever ensue from consuming the unhealthy, deadly foods which are rendered permissible under the Atkins diet that fall outside the salubrious food categories of fruits and vegetables. The only facet of the Atkins diet that is aligned with prudent dietary choices is the restriction of grains, cakes, wheat-based products, processed foods, processed oils, artificial sweeteners, juices, candies, ice creams, pastas, pastries, and cereals. In other words, the Atkins diet is essentially a low carbohydrate diet that places a emphasis on deriving calories from fat dense foods, such as dairy products, and protein dense foods, such as animal meats. However, even with these dietary restrictions imposed, avowed Atkins diet followers are preordained to succumb to inflammation and chronic diseases since the Atkins diet renders the consumption of a cornucopia of inflammatory, non-alkaline, disease promoting foods permissible. "The Atkins diet is a low carbohydrate diet, recommended by its proponents for weight loss. Proponents of this diet claim that you can lose weight while eating as much protein and fat as you want, as long as you avoid foods high in carbohydrates. The main reason why low carbohydrate diets are so effective for weight loss is that a reduction in carbohydrates and increased protein intake lead to reduced appetite, making you eat fewer calories without having to think about it" (Gunnars, 2018). Even though the Atkins diet, restricts the consumption of various unhealthy food groups, such as processed foods, the Atkins diet is still an eminently unhealthy, outright deadly, and highly disease promoting diet.Fortunately, the consumption of most synthetic, bastardized man made food products are not rendered permissible under the Atkins diet since these types of foods are carbohydrate dense and are often replete with sugars. Human beings under no circumstance should devour synthetic, bastardized man made food products, such as cereals, breads, noodles, pies, condiments, confectioneries, sauces, processed foods, baked foods, dumplings, fermented foods, sandwiches, potato chips, pretzels, pizzas, pastries, cakes, fast foods, candies, soups, snack foods, oils, and stews. These aforementioned products are not found in nature nor derived from the Earth. While some of these aforementioned products, such as sandwiches and soups may integrate some vegetables into them, they are still laced with ample disease promoting ingredients and therefore can be deadly for human consumption. Synthetic, bastardized man made processed foods for instance are devoid of nutritional value and are notorious for being laced with additives, pathogens, endocrine distributors, neurotoxins, noxious ingredients, sugars, animal byproducts, trans fats, and carcinogens. While some processed foods are far less detrimental to consume than others, they are all deemed unhealthy and are engineered to be addictive. Processed foods are highly inflammatory foods and are also not filling since they provide no real nutritional value. Processed foods are unsurprisingly linked to the development of ample chronic diseases, such as cardiovascular disease, diabetes, and cancer.

The Atkins diet is often erroneously touted as a healthy diet even though it is fraught with dietary issues that encompass rendering the consumption of ample unhealthy foods permissible, such as dairy products and animal products. Much to the chagrin of dieters, an exorbitant amount of non-alkaline, carcinogenic, acidic, pathogenic, cholesterol laced, endocrine distributive, inflammatory, and chronic disease promoting that are rendered permissible under the Atkins diet. The Atkins diet is unequivocally an unhealthy, deadly, and disease promoting diet for a myriad of reasons.

The Atkins diet renders the consumption of ample foods that profusely ravage the DNA, shorten the telomeres, unravel the chromosomes, comprise all facets of your health, elicit chronic diseases, draw forth severe inflammation, and that decrease your longevity rate permissible. In other words, nothing salubrious can ever ensue from consuming the unhealthy, deadly foods which are rendered permissible under the Atkins diet that fall outside the salubrious food categories of fruits and vegetables.

The only facet of the Atkins diet that is aligned with prudent dietary choices is the restriction of grains, cakes, wheat-based products, processed foods, processed oils, artificial sweeteners, juices, candies, ice creams, pastas, pastries, and cereals. In other words, the Atkins diet is essentially a low carbohydrate diet that places a emphasis on deriving calories from fat dense foods, such as dairy products, and protein dense foods, such as animal meats.

However, even with these dietary restrictions imposed, avowed Atkins diet followers are preordained to succumb to inflammation and chronic diseases since the Atkins diet renders the consumption of a cornucopia of inflammatory, non-alkaline, disease promoting foods permissible. "The Atkins diet is a low carbohydrate diet, recommended by its proponents for weight loss. Proponents of this diet claim that you can lose weight while eating as much protein and fat as you want, as long as you avoid foods high in carbohydrates. The main reason why low carbohydrate diets are so effective for weight loss is that a reduction in carbohydrates and increased protein intake lead to reduced appetite, making you eat fewer calories without having to think about it" (Gunnars, 2018). Even though the Atkins diet, restricts the consumption of various unhealthy food groups, such as processed foods, the Atkins diet is still an eminently unhealthy, outright deadly, and highly disease promoting diet.

Fortunately, the consumption of most synthetic, bastardized man made food products are not rendered permissible under the Atkins diet since these types of foods are carbohydrate dense and are often replete with sugars. Human beings under no circumstance should devour synthetic, bastardized man made food products, such as cereals, breads, noodles, pies, condiments, confectioneries, sauces, processed foods, baked foods, dumplings, fermented foods, sandwiches, potato chips, pretzels, pizzas, pastries, cakes, fast foods, candies, soups, snack foods, oils, and stews. These aforementioned products are not found in nature nor derived from the Earth. While some of these aforementioned products, such as sandwiches and soups may integrate some vegetables into them, they are still laced with ample disease promoting ingredients and therefore can be deadly for human consumption.

Synthetic, bastardized man made processed foods for instance are devoid of nutritional value and are notorious for being laced with additives, pathogens, endocrine distributors, neurotoxins, noxious ingredients, sugars, animal byproducts, trans fats, and carcinogens. While some processed foods are far less detrimental to consume than others, they are all deemed unhealthy and are engineered to be addictive. Processed foods are highly inflammatory foods and are also not filling since they provide no real nutritional value. Processed foods are unsurprisingly linked to the development of ample chronic diseases, such as cardiovascular disease, diabetes, and cancer.

The consumption of these synthetic, bastardized man made food products leads to a host of health issues beyond inflammation that are not limited to free radical damage, high blood pressure, high blood sugar levels, high LDL cholesterol levels, insulin resistance, clogged arteries, nutritional deficiencies, hormone imbalances, digestive distress, migraines, constipation, accelerated aging, increased stress, obesity, decreased testosterone levels, telomere shortening, and other calamitous health issues.

Consuming even a minor amount of ultra-processed foods overtime can be eminently detrimental to your health. "In an observational study by JAMA Internal Medicine, almost 45,000 adults ages 45 and older completed several dietary assessments over a two-year period. On average, ultra-processed foods made up only about 15% of their daily diet as measured in grams. Ultra-processed food was defined as ready-to-eat and microwaveable foods, such as bread, breakfast cereals, instant noodles, chicken or fish nuggets, chocolate bars and candies, chips, and artificially sweetened beverages" ("Eating more ultra-processed," 2019). The results of the study after a nine year period were devastatingly bleak for processed food lovers.

Unfortunately, for the processed food lovers, "the researchers found a direct statistical connection between higher intake of ultra-processed food and a higher risk of early death from all causes, especially cancers and cardiovascular disease. Several factors might explain the connection, according to the researchers. Ultra-processed foods often have fewer nutrients than unprocessed foods, and they contain higher amounts of sugar, salt, saturated fat, and food additives, all of which are associated with an increased risk for chronic diseases" ("Eating more ultra-processed," 2019). It is no surprise that synthetic, bastardized man made food products have garnered a terrible reputation over the years and are deemed the epitome of junk food since they always belong in the trash and never in the human body. Even extra virgin oils that mistakenly believed to be healthy should also be relegated to the trash since they are highly oxidized products and are therefore not fit for human consumption.

As frugivores, humans were not designed to eat animal products nor synthetic, bastardized man made food products. The consumption of inflammatory, disease promoting, carcinogenic, non-alkaline animal products and synthetic, bastardized man made food products can be lethal to the individual's health in all facets.

Even with the restriction of most synthetic, bastardized man made food products that are replete with sugars and carbohydrates, the Atkins diet is still an eminently unhealthy, deadly dietary regimen to follow. The benefits of the Atkins diet, such as avoiding consuming grains and ample synthetic man made food products, are preponderantly outweighed by its myriad of deleterious downsides, such as promoting the consumption of animal products and dairy products. Animal products are notorious for being highly inflammatory, disease promoting products which are lethal for human consumption.

First and foremost, under the Atkins diet, the consumption of animal products, including animal carcasses and animal byproducts is rendered permissible. It is of utmost importance that you never consume any type of animal products, such as fish, beef, pork, hamburgers, poultry, hot dogs, sausages, lard, shellfish, shrimp, lobster, and any other types of deleterious animal products. These animal products are not meant to ever be consumed by humans since human beings have the innate anatomy of a fruigovore and not a carnivore. As frugivores with long intestines and high PH levels, human beings will not be able to efficaciously digest these lethal animal products without it being of dire consequence to their overall health.

Consumption of these deadly animal products creates a deleterious recipe for not only acute inflammation and the cultivation of every major life threatening chronic disease, but also elicit free radical damage, high blood pressure, high blood sugar levels, high LDL cholesterol levels, insulin resistance, clogged arteries, nutritional deficiencies, hormone imbalances, digestive distress, migraines, constipation, accelerated aging, increased stress, high mercury levels, obesity, and other calamitous issues. The havoc that animal proteins, animal fats, animal secretions, and animal byproducts can wreak on the individual's overall health and longevity should not be underestimated.

For instance, "one study conducted by the Harvard School of Public Health in 2014 found that one serving a day of red meat in adolescence or early adulthood had a 22% higher risk of perimenopausal breast cancer. Each serving per day led to a 13% higher risk of breast cancer overall" (Sunday, 2018). Animal meat and red meat are lethal, acidic, carcinogenic, pathogenic, non-alkaline products that not only ravage DNA and severely undermine your overall health, but also help draw forth the conditions inside your body for a tumor to rapidly proliferate and metastasize to other vital organs.

The deleterious health problems that the consumption of animal products draws forth extends far beyond just elicit cancer inside the body. For example, "the National Cancer Institute of

Maryland conducted the largest study so far to link both processed and unprocessed meat to an increase in death rates from nine diseases. These include heart disease, stroke, diabetes, Alzheimer's and lung disease" (Sunday, 2018). The ramifications of consuming animal carcasses, animal byproducts, and animal secretions are always adverse for human beings since it will veritably comprise every facet of their health.

Second, the Atkins diet renders the consumption of dairy products permissible. Dairy products can include cheeses, yogurts, and milk. Dairy products are deadly products for humans to consume and should never be devoured. Consumption of these types of dairy based animal products not only can draw forth acute inflammation, but can also elicit a deleterious recipe for the cultivation of every major life threatening chronic disease.

Just like other types of animal products, such as animal carcasses, red meat, and fish products, these dairy based animal products also cause a myriad of dire health issues including, free radical damage, high blood pressure, high blood sugar levels, high LDL cholesterol levels, insulin resistance, clogged arteries, nutritional deficiencies, hormone imbalances, digestive distress, migraines, constipation, accelerated aging, increased stress, obesity, decreased testosterone levels, and other calamitous issues. In other words, nothing fruitful can transpire from tainting your body with dairy based animal products nor egg based animal products.

For instance, the consumption of cow milk can play a major role in the development of a seemingly irreversible disease, type 1 diabetes. "Multiple large-scale studies have identified an association between cow's milk consumption and increased prevalence of type 1 diabetes. One such study found that cows' milk may contain a triggering factor for the development of IDDM, and another found that early cow's milk exposure may be an important determinant of subsequent type 1 diabetes and may increase the risk approximately 1.5 times. Moreover, as with type 1 diabetes, numerous studies have reported that cow's milk consumption may be a significant risk factor for also developing Multiple Sclerosis" (Ochoa, 2016).

Dairy products are also replete with IGF-1, "a hormone that promotes cell growth and division in both normal and cancer cells" (Ochoa, 2016). Moreover, dairy product also contain ample foodborne pathogens, microorganisms, organochlorine pesticides, antibiotic residues (Ochoa, 2016), endocrine distributors, neurotoxins, and carcinogens.

For instance, "Salmonella, Listeria, and E. coli are some of the more common foodborne outbreaks associated with dairy. Just last year, for example, three people tragically died from Listeria infections linked to Blue Bell Ice Cream (prompting a large-scale recall by Blue Bell Creameries)" (Ochoa, 2016). Dairy products are so deadly that the consumption of animal secretion products, such as ice cream, can deprive you of your life.

Dairy products are also detrimental to bone health. "Numerous large-scale studies have found that consuming dairy can comprise bone health. In fact, there is substantial data linking higher milk intake with significantly increased risk of bone fractures. The high animal protein content of dairy can induce acidosis from its high proportion of sulfur-containing amino acids, which in turn leads to the body compensating by leaching calcium from the bones to help neutralize the increased acidity. Overtime, all of this can have an eminently deleterious effect on bone health" (Ochoa, 2016). It is preponderantly ill-advised to ever consume any type of animal products, including dairy products and egg products, since the repercussions of consuming disease promoting foods can be life threatening.

Third, much to the dismay of the health conscious individual, the Atkins diet promotes the consumption of foods fraught with anti-nutrients that can comprise gut health and elicit other health issues. While the Atkins diet restricts the consumption of grains and legumes, it still encourages the consumption of nuts and seeds which unfortunately are laced with anti-nutrients.

It is incumbent to always desist from consuming whole grains, refined grains, legumes, nuts, and seeds if you desire to optimize your health and avert succumbing to dire health issues, such as comprising your gut health. It is ill-advised to consume whole grains, refined grains, legumes, nuts, and seeds primarily because they are eminently taxing on the digestive system and are laced with anti-nutrients. For instance, the phytates and phytic acid in whole grains, seeds, and legumes can inhibit or minimize the absorption of certain minerals, such as iron, calcium, and zinc. Moreover, the consumption of these aforementioned protein dense plant based food groups can potentially decimate the microvilli overtime and also wreak havoc on the gut lining. The microvilli play a critical role in allowing the small intestine to absorb vital nutrients, vitamins, and minerals.

The human body does not have the anatomy to efficaciously break down the complex amino acids found in grains, legumes, nuts, and seeds. Moreover, the body is not designed to seamlessly digest these aforementioned protein dense plant based foods. These food groups also contain lectins, a plant based protein which acts as a natural pesticide that can be extremely harmful to the body and gut health overtime. The types of lectins infamous for eliciting health problems are prolamins and agglutinins.

During a meal, the body churns out enzymes in order to break down proteins into amino acids. However, when inhibited by the chemicals within seeds, the enzymes cannot perform this essential task which ultimately causes a chain reaction. Once a chain reaction has transpired, your vessel subsequently produces even more enzymes. During this strenuousness digestive process, the body's nutrients are being exhausted while you in return do not assimilate the incoming nutrients. If this process transpires daily then an overabundance of digestive enzymes in the gut will not only ravage the gut lining, but will also elicit leaky gut syndrome.

Moreover, as the intestinal tract amasses an overabundance of partially digested foods, such as partially digested grains, there is an oversupply of food for the body's bacteria. This can ultimately cause a bacteria imbalance to transpire within the intestinal tract and lead to a variety of other calamitous health issues from bacterial overgrowth, such as the outright severing of the gut lining (Myers, n.d.).

"The gut is designed to only be slightly permeable. The ability for some substances to pass through the gut lining is an essential function of our bodies, allowing us to absorb nutrients from our food, fight infection, and assemble the proteins and enzymes that are necessary for life. However, the gut can become hyperpermeable, and this can lead to autoimmunity. Because they are not completely digested, grains, pseudograins, and legumes pass through the gut barrier intact. This helps to increase the permeability of the gut barrier a) by damaging the cells that line the gut and b) by causing an inflammatory response once outside the gut. A cycle then begins where the body responds to the grain particles with inflammation, which then damages the gut lining, which in turn becomes even more permeable, allowing more undigested food, toxins, and bacteria to leak out. Your body can confuse these foreign 'invaders' with your own tissues – a process known as molecular mimicry. Soon, the immune response gets out of control and begins to affect more tissues and systems within the body, and autoimmunity results" (Myers, n.d.).

Moreover, "grains, pseudograins, and legumes are not nutrient-dense foods, and they can actually prevent you from absorbing the amino acids you need for a healthy immune system. Even grain varieties that are promoted as wheat-free alternatives are just as devoid of nutrients. It is much better to replace these inflammatory foods with healthier choices such as sweet potato, squash, and dark leafy greens" (Myers, n.d.).

As frugivores, whole grains, seeds, nuts, and legumes are unequally deadly for human consumption, primarily because they not only comprise the small intestine's ability to absorb nutrients by wreaking havoc against the microvilli with their complex amino acids and anti-nutrients, but also decimate the body's gut lining and lead to a host of undesirable health issues. These inflammatory foods groups should never be eaten and should be replaced with nutrient dense fruits and vegetables characterized by high levels of alkalinity that also have low glycemic loads, such as avocados and zucchini.

In order to optimize all facets of health, it is salient that whole grains, seeds, nuts, and legumes are never incorporated into your diet. Even the vegan diet renders the incorporation of inflammatory food groups that elicit dire long term health complications, such as comprised gut health and malabsorption issues, permissible and is therefore, unequivocally, also not a healthy dietary regimen to follow even though it is a vast improvement over the Atkins diet.

Fourth, the Atkins diet promotes the consumption of egg products. Humans should always desist from consuming any type of egg products, such as eggnog, mayonnaise, and custard. Egg products induce free radical damage, high blood pressure, high LDL cholesterol levels, insulin resistance, clogged arteries, hormone imbalances, digestive distress, migraines, constipation, accelerated aging, increased stress, obesity, decreased testosterone levels, telomere shortening, and other calamitous health issues. The human body is not designed to efficaciously digest egg products and the ramifications of doing so can be eminently dire.

After performing an "analysis of six previous studies that included nearly 30,000 Americans, researchers ascertained that eating just half an egg a day was linked to a 6%-8% increased risk of having a heart attack, stroke, or early death over the course of the study, compared to someone who did not eat eggs. Moreover, the more eggs a person ate, the more those risks increased. People in the study who averaged an egg every day saw their risk of a heart-related event such as a heart attack or stroke increase by 12% compared to someone who did not consume eggs. Those who averaged two eggs every day had a 24% increased risk of heart-related events. Additionally, researchers found similarly increased risks for people who ate processed and unprocessed red meat" ("Are Eggs The," 2019). In other words, eating eggs is not only lethal to your overall health, but is practically equivalent to consuming red meat in terms of its effect on your health.

Nothing salubrious can ensue from eating egg products and the outcome of following an unhealthy, deadly diet that renders ample unhealthy food groups permissible, such as dairy products and egg products, vindicates why the Atkins diet should never be followed. The outcome of embracing a Atkins diet will be perilous to every facet of your health since it does not restrict the consumption of all unhealthy, deadly food groups. While the benefits of restricting grains and ample synthetic man made foods from your diet are a step in the right direction for increasing your longevity rate, the Atkins diet is still not restrictive enough for allowing the individual to preempt succumbing to inflammation and chronic diseases. The Atkins diet renders the consumption of a myriad of unhealthy, inflammatory, and chronic disease promoting foods permissible which ultimately renders it a perilous and unhealthy dietary regimen to follow.

Making poor dietary choices cannot only cause chronic inflammation, but can also easily comprise your overall health since the deleterious outcome of eating deadly foods will not only comprise every facet of your health, but will also eventually elicit a chronic disease that will deprive you of your life. Moreover, poor dietary choices will not only render your body distressed, but will also lead to telomere shortening, DNA damage, cancer cell proliferation, free radical damage, high blood pressure, high blood sugar levels, high LDL cholesterol levels, insulin resistance, clogged arteries, nutritional deficiencies, hormone imbalances, digestive distress, migraines, constipation, accelerated aging, increased stress, obesity, decreased testosterone levels, high mercury levels, chronic inflammation, and other calamitous health issues. In a distressed state, the body cannot function optimally and can only sustain so much hardship, malnourishment, and complications that eventually lead to its organs shutting down.

Making imprudent dietary disease by consuming deadly foods can render the body disease ridden, severely inflamed, and severely impaired. For instance, "a cancer that grows in part of the digestive system can block it, or partly block it. This causes foods to not be able to go through the intestines. The nutrients and calories you need cannot be absorbed" ("How can cancer," 2014) when this transpire.

Moreover, "a cancer that has spread to the liver or bones can upset the body's chemical balance. The liver is the chemical factory of the body. It carries out many tasks and is very important in maintaining the balance of body chemicals. It can be life threatening if this chemical balance cannot be corrected"

("How can cancer," 2014). Chronic diseases are simply the culmination of the individual having accrued making poor dietary choices throughout their life. Poor dietary choices can easily truncate someone's life by decades and drastically increase their mortality rate since the body has a limit to its resilience and cannot mend itself properly when it is unremittingly under a state of distress from poor dietary decisions that severely undermine its innate healing capabilities. Chronic inflammation induced from making poor dietary choices is an experience that is always agonizing which denotes that the body is under a state of severe distress.

The individual should consume only foods subsumed under a heart healthy, anticancer, nutrient dense, antioxidant rich, anti-inflammatory, alkaline, raw fruitarian diet for the prospect of enhancing their health and prolonging their life. In spite of its wealth of health benefits it offers, virtually all individuals lack the self-discipline to embrace a heart healthy, anticancer, nutrient dense, antioxidant rich, anti-inflammatory, alkaline, raw fruitarian diet. Fortunately, for raw fruitarians, alkaline fruits and vegetables are succulent, scrumptious, delectable, savory, palatable, flavorful, delicious, and appreciating. Alkaline Fruits and vegetables have natural flavors and never need any additives nor any noxious ingredients to ever be added to them to taste exquisite.

There are ample easy to prepare, appetizing healthy food recipes that can serve as a robust panacea for preventing deadly chronic diseases, such as cardiovascular disease and cancer, and can also play a salient role in improving your health and prolonging your life due to their ample medicinal properties. These easy to prepare, scrumptious healthy food recipes are subsumed under a heart healthy, anticancer, nutrient dense, antioxidant rich, anti-inflammatory, alkaline, raw fruitarian diet. Foods apart of these healthy food recipes are fruits and vegetables that are characterized by high levels of alkalinity that also bear a low glycemic load. Moreover, these healthy food recipes are also chalk-full of phytonutrients, macronutrients, micronutrients, antioxidants, vitamins, minerals, digestive enzymes, fiber, anticancer properties, and other salubrious compounds. These easy to prepare robustly healthy food recipes draw forth succulent, scrumptious, delectable, savory, palatable, flavorful, appetizing, delicious, sapid, and nourishing meals that unequivocally will eminently stimulate your taste buds.

First and foremost, one ineffably healthy, appetizing food recipe that is easy to prepare entails submerging frozen cauliflower in water and subsequently eating the thawed out cauliflower florets with black olives. You can also add coarse sea salt or Pink Himalayan salt to further augment the flavor profile of the meal. The saltiness of the meal, sulfur-like flavor of the cauliflower, and nutty taste of the black olives truly renders this meal sensation to all your taste buds. The frozen cauliflower vastly trumps the non-frozen cauliflower in terms of its overall flavor profile since frozen food is far more nutrient dense than refrigerated food that has succumbed to oxidation.

Second, another inexplicably healthy, appetizing food recipe that is easy to prepare involves eating avocados in tandem with black olives. You can also add coarse sea salt or Pink Himalayan salt to further accentuate the salty flavor facet of the meal. The saltiness of the black olives, the creaminess of the avocados, and the nutty taste of these fat dense fruits truly renders this meal exquisite to all your taste buds, especially if the avocados have ripened properly and are not in a distressed state.

Third, another extraordinary appetizing, healthy food recipe that is easy to prepare involves eating a raw iceberg lettuce head in conjunction with tomatoes and sea salt. You can alternatively profusely add Pink Himalayan salt to the meal in lieu of the addition of coarse sea salt to the meal. The mild flavor of the lettuce head renders the savoriness of the tomatoes eminently delectable and more palatable. Moreover, the iceberg lettuce head also serves as a versatile, staple vegetable for the meal. This ultimately allows other unique healthy food recipes to be developed which expand upon the health food recipe for the meal. In other words, you can expand upon the aforementioned healthy recipe of eating a raw iceberg lettuce head in conjunction with tomatoes and sea salt in order to develop your own vegan salad that panders to your loftiest vegan meal dreams.

Fourth, another salubrious, appetizing food recipe that is easy to prepare entails procuring mini cucumbers or seedless cucumbers and profusely sprinkling them with sea salt or Pink Himalayan salt to revolutionize the flavor profile of the meal. This will render the formerly tasteless mini cucumber into your own version of salty alkaline vegan pickles that you can prepare in seconds without the need for a brine nor anything deem unhealthy to bring the salty, alkaline vegan pickles to fruition that can be prepared in mere seconds with just two simple ingredients, mini cucumbers and sea salt.

Fifth, another robustly healthy, appetizing food recipe that is easy to prepare involves eating brussel sprouts in conjunction with black olives and sea salt. You can also profusely add coarse Pink Himalayan salt instead of sea salt to the meal in order to further enhance the salty facet of the meal's flavor profile. The bitter flavor of the brussel sprouts contrasts eminently well with the nutty taste of the black olive. This ultimately allow the flavor profile of the black olives to be profoundly accentuated. Moreover, the meal's flavor profile becomes even more of a distinguishable salty, nutty, fatty, and piquant meal with the addition of Pink Himalayan salt to the black olives and brussel sprouts.

Reaping maximum pleasure out of these highly appetizing, robustly healthy food recipes that are easy to prepare entails consuming all the ingredients per bite that are associated with their respective healthy food recipes. For instance, if you followed the first robustly healthy food recipe that is easy to prepare then this would simply entail each bite of the meal being comprised of an olive, a piece of cauliflower, and some sea salt. You can provide maximum stimuli to your taste palate when each bite maximizes the amount of the recipe's ingredients you can taste and is never limited to experiencing only a single ingredient.

Other noteworthy, appetizing healthy food recipes that draw forth succulent, scrumptious, delectable, savory, palatable, flavorful, appreciating meals that capitalize on utilize sea salt to augment the flavor profiles of vegetables or mushrooms encompass profusely sprinkling sea salt onto hearts of palm, profusely sprinkling sea salt onto seaweed, profusely sprinkling sea salt onto shiitake mushrooms, profusely sprinkling sea salt onto beets, profusely sprinkling sea salt onto zucchini. These aforementioned vegetables and the shiitake mushrooms have simple flavor profiles that are eminently augmented by the addition of sea salt. These aforementioned easy healthy food recipes can be prepared in seconds and provide affordable meal options for individuals to follow since they are limited to only 2 ingredients. Sea salt complements these aforementioned foods and profoundly evolves the flavor profiles of these foods to an ineffably unprecedented degree.

These easy to prepare, appetizing healthy food recipes are comprised of healthy ingredients that stave off diseases and have ample medicinal properties. Embracing following only healthy food recipes when preparing meals will have bearing on allowing you to enhance your overall health and prolong your life, especially if the meals are only comprised of only fruits and vegetables. Fruits and vegetables are considered the only two healthy food groups and are chalk-full of phytonutrients, macronutrients, micronutrients, antioxidants, vitamins, minerals, digestive enzymes, fiber, anticancer properties, and other salubrious compounds.

There are ample foods that the individual should consume in order to substantially reduce risks for succumbing to a deadly chronic disease. The foods that the individual should profusely consume are subsumed under a heart healthy, anticancer, nutrient dense, antioxidant rich, anti-inflammatory, alkaline, raw fruitarian foods. In order to preclude perilous chronic disease, the individual should eat only fruits and vegetables that are characterized by high levels of alkalinity that also have a low glycemic load.

A vast variety of nutrient dense, anticancer, alkaline fruits and vegetables can play a salient role in revitalizing, nourishing, and empowering the individual so that his it is highly unlikely that he will ever succumb to a major chronic disease, such as cancer, type 2 diabetes, lung disease, or cardiovascular disease. Ideally, the individual should profusely consume heart healthy, anticancer, nutrient dense, antioxidant rich, anti-inflammatory, alkaline, raw fruitarian foods.

Some of the ample nutrient fruits to choose from encompass avocados, olives, durian, grapes, grapefruits, peppers, cranberries, cherries, apricots, tomatoes, mangoes, oranges, pineapples, kiwis, strawberries, pears, cucumbers, papayas, guavas, nectarines, dragon fruit, and peaches. These aforementioned fruits are chalk-full of phytonutrients, macronutrients, micronutrients, antioxidants, vitamins, minerals, digestive enzymes, fiber, and other salubrious anticancer compounds. There medicinal properties and anticancer properties render them potent elixirs of life. They also play a vital role in optimizing the individual's overall health and prolonging their lifespan. It is paramount for the individual to only consume anticancer, heart healthy, nutrient dense, antioxidant rich, anti-inflammatory, alkaline, raw fruitarian foods if he is keen on preempting contracting a deadly chronic disease, such as cancer.

"Citrus fruits for instance, such as orange, grapefruits, lime, and lemon" (Gamble, 2015), can have tremendous bearing on helping to preventing chronic diseases, such as Alzheimer's disease and lung disease. Moreover, "citrus fruits are considered alkaline fruits" (Gamble, 2015) since they leave an alkaline residue in the body post being digested. Additionally, "their alkaline nature combined with their citrus compounds can also help prevent kidney stones" (Gamble, 2015) which is all the more reason why the individual should be keen on consuming ample citrus fruits.

It is also incumbent to assimilate adequate levels of Vitamin D from plant based sources. "Low levels of vitamin D increase your risk of risk." (Oberst, 2017). In other words, low levels of vitamin D may increase your chances of developing lethal chronic diseases. For instance, "according to one study, low levels of vitamin D doubled the risk of stroke in Caucasians" (Oberst, 2017). Moreover, "low levels of vitamin D have been linked to increased risk of asthma attacks in children and adults"("Asthma and Nutrition," 2018). You can increase your vitamin D levels by consuming vegan vitamin D3 supplements. "Vitamin D plays an important role in boosting immune system responses and helps to reduce airway inflammation" ("Asthma and Nutrition," 2018). It is critical to maintain a healthy BMI, attain optimal sleep, and desist from ever consuming chronic disease causing foods so that you can further substantially decrease the risk of succumbing to deadly maladies.

Moreover, vegetables are also rendered permissible under the anticancer, heart healthy, nutrient dense, antioxidant rich, anti-inflammatory, alkaline, raw fruitarian diet.. Some of the cornucopia of healthy vegetables encompass garlic, onions, broccoli, brussel sprouts, cauliflower, collard, bok choy, carrots, artichokes, seaweed, hearts of palm, watercress, zucchini, yellow squash, kale, arugula, turnips, radishes, and cabbage. These aforementioned vegetables are also chalk-full of phytonutrients, macronutrients, micronutrients, antioxidants, vitamins, minerals, digestive enzymes, fiber, anticancer properties, and other salubrious compounds. Moreover, "according to studies led by Harvard researchers, greens turned out to be associated with the strongest protection against major chronic diseases, including a 20% reduction for strokes and heart disease for every additional serving" (Oberst, 2017).

Consumption of only heart healthy, anticancer, antioxidant rich, anti-inflammatory, alkaline, fruits and vegetables coupled with the abstinence of anything deem unhealthy, non-alkaline, insalubrious, carcinogenic, or toxin can play a salient role in mitigating risks of succumbing to a chronic disease. Man's utmost potent natural panacea for warding off chronic diseases is perhaps a raw fruitarian diet coupled with prolonged fasting that allows the individual to reap the myriad of salubrious benefits that ensue from attaining an alkaline body.

Before you undergo a prolonged fast, you want to ensure that you have a healthy BMI of well above 18.5, have recently consumed a copious amount of nutrient dense fruits and vegetables to nourish the vessel, are eminently hydrated, and do not have to do anything too physical intense amid this fasting period. I personally attempt to eat 5,000-20,000 calories per meal before undergoing a prolonged fast.

Robustly healthy fruits and vegetables are the optimal panacea for preventing chronic diseases since they not only promote optimal lung health, optimal cognitive health, optimal artery health, optimal blood flow, optimal kidney health, optimal urinary tract health, optimal vascular health, optimal blood sugar health, enhanced insulin sensitivity, healthy cholesterol levels, healthy blood pressure levels, healthy weight levels, but also help elicit an alkaline microcosm in the body in addition to providing other benefits, such as preventing blood clots, starving off free radical damage, attenuating inflammation derived from the air passageways, and preempting exorbitant plaque buildup in the arteries and brain. Moreover, it is also imperative that you consume vegan supplements from plant based sources of nutrients and vitamins that your diet may be devoid of, such as Vitamin B12, Nascent Iodine, and Vitamin D3, to ensure that your body has all the requisite nutrients it needs to attain robust, vigorous health.

It is paramount to drink a copious amount of distilled water as deemed necessary in order stay hydrated and discharge mineral waste from the body. Drinking distilled water can also bolster lung health, mental acuity, can help facilitate the process of expunging toxins from the brain and even mucus from the lungs. A lack of water for instance can also cause the blood to thicken, can hamper your brain's reaction times, and can even increase your chances of succumbing to a stroke. For instance, "studies have even shown that people who are afflicted with heart disease and/or have previously suffered a stroke can drastically reduce their risk of a future, fatal stroke by half just by keeping properly hydrated" ("Water and Stroke," n.d.)." 'Staying well hydrated by taking in fluids throughout the day helps keep the mucosal linings in the lungs thin. This thinner lining helps the lungs function better' "("8 Tips for," n.d.).

The repercussions of being dehydrated can be fatal which is why it is eminently important to stay hydrated. Fruits and vegetables are water rich foods and can play a salient role in helping to keep the body hydrated.

"Eating foods that are high in antioxidants like vitamins C and E is a wonderful natural way to eliminate free radicals from your body. In a similar way, scientists believe that a vast intake of fruits and vegetable can even protect against oxidative stress in the lungs and even memory loss. Vitamin C for instance has even been shown to reduce your risk of Alzheimer's disease by 20% when taken in tandem with vitamin E" ("Pillar 1: Diet," n.d.). The profuse consumption of distilled water, citrus fruits, magnesium rich vegetables, Vitamin C rich fruits, potassium rich fruits, and

Vitamin E rich fruits can also play a pivotal role in helping to prevent disease.

Easily optimizing your overall health and maximizing your longevity rate goes far beyond attaining an alkaline body from following a nutrient dense, anti-inflammatory, antioxidant rich, anticancer, raw fruitarian diet comprised of foods characterized by high levels of alkalinity that have low glycemic loads. Partaking in prolonged fasting, maintaining healthy social circles, engaging in heart healthy exercises daily, attaining ample REM sleep, participating in stress alleviating activities daily, minimizing time spend towards sedentariness, minimizing exposure to second hand smoke and other deleterious compounds, and living a fulfilling life to its fullest in which you demonstrate unconditional love and forgiveness towards everyone are presumably key factors for allowing you to optimize your health and maximize your longevity rate. Some of the numerous nutrient dense, alkaline fruits and vegetables foods that promote longevity encompass avocados, onions, olives, garlic, tomatoes, cherries, grapes, broccoli, brussel sprouts, and cabbage (Fuhrman, 2018). Additionally, with their anti-inflammatory proprieties and other robust health benefits, spices such as ginger, turmeric, black pepper, and sea salt, can presumably help reverse the signs of aging, prolong life, and promote optimal health. Dietary choices perhaps have the utmost bearing of all the life style factors on influencing your future health and longevity rate.

Heart healthy, nutrient dense, antioxidant rich, anti-inflammatory, alkaline, raw fruits and vegetables are truly the divine elixirs of life with all their medicinal properties and anticancer properties. For instance, it is reasonable to conclude that the elixir for curing a chronic disease, such as cancer, may not lie in any man made pill. Rather, reversing and curing cancer may entail creating an alkaline microcosm in your body, starving cancer cells by depriving them of access to glucose, resetting your immune system on a weekly basis; and reaping the ample health benefits prolonged fasting, ketosis, autophagy, and the consumption of nutrient dense, alkaline fruits and vegetables has to offer.

The elixir for reversing and curing cancer may presumably lie in creating all the requisite conditions within an alkaline microcosm of an eminently nourished body in order to ultimately profusely exploit and optimize its innate, divine healing mechanisms so that it can eliminate cancer cells far more efficaciously and rapidly than ever thought possible. Anticancer, alkaline, anti-inflammatory, nutrient dense, raw fruits and vegetables can play a salient role in allowing the body to more efficaciously eliminate cancer cells since they not only help elicit an alkaline microcosm in the body, but also play a pivotal role in optimizing overall health. It is critical for the body to not be in a distressed state so that it can begin to more potently innately mend itself from aliments and maladies. Moreover, as mentioned previously, it is also imperative that you consume vegan supplements from plant based sources of nutrients and vitamins that your diet may be devoid of, such as Vitamin B12, Nascent Iodine, and Vitamin D3, to ensure that your body has all the requisite nutrients it needs to attain robust, vigorous health.

As fruitful as the endeavor of conducting cancer research may sound, it is unequivocally a sheer and utter waste of money. A man made medication will never be able to cure a stage 4 tumor and all the money spent on this counter productive endeavor has been completely squandered on arguably unavailing research activities. Even though reversing and curing chronic diseases may simply lie in embracing a raw fruitarian diet coupled with prolonged fasting, it is highly unlikely that this panacea will ever become mainstream and prevalent. Most people do not have the self-discipline to embrace prolonged fasting nor can even simply omit carcinogenic, non-alkaline, acidic, pathogenic, oxidized, cholesterol laced products from their diet which ravage their DNA, wreak havoc against their immune system, cause a host of dire health issues, promote chronic diseases, and ultimately shorten their telomeres. "We also need to recognize that the more than $90 billion spent in pursuit of a cure has not achieved the most effective 'cure' of all, preventing the disease to begin with. Cancer's role in one out of every four deaths in the country remains a haunting statistic" (Cuomo, 2012).

The crux of the issue with the cancer research investment lies in the fact that medications just provide systematic relief and do not remedy the root cause of a disease. This is why the tumors can persist and proliferate even when cancer medications are profusely consumed. Someone cannot expect a medication that may offer systematic relief and possibly mask the symptoms to remedy the cancer when the patient is still imprudently doing everything in their purview to create all the conditions needed for the tumor to thrive, prosper, flourish, and proliferate in an acidic environment. In other words, when you are incessantly creating the requisite conditions to further cultivate a chronic disease in your already tainted vessel, you cannot expect a man made medication to negate all these persisting issues as the ailing valetudinarian continues to partake in a chronic disease promoting lifestyle by imprudently embracing not only a deleterious dietary regimen, but also other insalubrious lifestyle decisions as well.

The research to concoct a man made medication for the prospect of curing cancer will also ultimately culminate in being a fruitless endeavor since no man made medication will likely ever be potent enough to negate the ramifications of these persisting chronic disease promoting lifestyle decisions that the cancer positive patient continues to incessantly pursue. Man made medications can also bare dire side effects against the organs and can even further exacerbate health. Unlike alkaline fruits, these man made medications are not something that the vessel is designed to efficaciously process. As a devolved, maladaptive species, we do not have the capability to innately alter our anatomy for our vessels to able to efficaciously process man made medications without experiencing possible calamitous side effects against the organs, such as possible heart problems and lung problems.

Mutations that transpire from poor lifestyle choices are also always adverse and unfortunately bastardize the original genetic code. Contrary to the common misconception, genetic mutations are never beneficial. Cancer cells for instance are simply mutated cell and they are eminently unresponsive to the various cell cycle control signals Attaining symptomatic relief through made made medications is unfortunately not conducive to actually curing a chronic disease.

For someone to have a chance of reversing a chronic disease, they need to not only stop the root cause of the disease and completely desist from ever making chronic disease promoting lifestyle choices, but also need to create the conditions conducive to optimizing the body's innate divine healing mechanics. In a cause and effect simulation, you cannot expect a cause to not elicit an effect. In other words, meteorically speaking, someone cannot expect to keep eating their cake without health consequences by consuming a man made medication for the prospect of fully negating or reversing the ensuing health issues caused by continual chronic disease promoting dietary choices that the individual still always imprudently pursues. Man made medications will clearly never be able to cure the cancer of a cancer positive patient who continues to imprudently embrace cancer promoting dietary decisions and insalubrious lifestyle decisions needed for the tumor to thrive, prosper, flourish, and relentlessly metastasize to other organs. It is unfortunate that people would rather eat unsavory, repulsive, chronic disease promotion foods rather than prolong their lives and optimize their health by embracing a nutrient dense, anti-inflammatory, antioxidant rich, anticancer, heart healthy, alkaline, raw fruitarian diet that has the potential to reverse chronic maladies, such as cancer, heart disease, and type 2 diabetes, and is also only limited to fruits and vegetables as food options coupled with capitalizing on the profound health benefits of undergoing prolonged fasting,

As previously mentioned, it is reasonable to conclude that man's utmost potent natural panacea for warding off cancer is perhaps a raw fruitarian diet coupled with prolonged fasting that allows the individual to reap the salubrious benefits that ensue from attaining an alkaline body. By creating an alkaline microcosm in your body, by starving the cancer cells by depriving them of access to glucose, by being able to reset your immune system on a weekly basis, and by being able to avail yourself of the health benefits of nutrient dense fruits and vegetables, prolonged fasting, ketosis, and autophagy, it is reasonable to conclude that the elixir for curing cancer may not lie in any man made pill. Rather, the elixir for prevent or curing cancer may however lie in creating all the requisite conditions in an alkaline microcosm of an eminently nourished body to ultimately profusely exploit and optimize its innate, divine healing mechanisms so that it can eliminate cancer cells far more efficaciously and rapidly than ever presumed possible.

Curing cancer may simply lie in embracing a raw fruitarian diet coupled with prolonged fasting. By eating fruits and vegetables that are characterized by high levels of alkalinity that also have a low glycemic load, such as avocados and cauliflower, you not only attain an alkaline body with a blood pH level above 7.35, but can also create a microcosm in your body that also preempts the formation of tumors and fatty plaque build up in the arteries, especially when combined with the power of prolonged fasting. "Dr. Ornish and colleagues conducted a study with cancer patients and found that the progression of prostate cancer could be reversed with a plant-based diet and other healthy lifestyle behaviors. After eating healthy, their own bodies were able to somehow reprogram the cancer cells, forcing them into early retirement. Nothing appears to kick more cancer tush than a plant-based diet. Even 5,000 hours in the gym was no match for the benefits of a plant-based diet" ("Kick Cancer with", n.d.) when it came to terminating cancer cells. By following a nutrient dense, anti-inflammatory, antioxidant rich, anticancer, raw fruitarian comprised of only fruits and vegetables, you are able to create the conditions to not only attain an alkaline body with a blood pH level above 7.35 which creates an anti-cancer microcosm, but also is associated with a substantially lower circulating IGF-1 level. IGF-1, also known as "insulin-like growth factor 1, is a cancer-promoting growth hormone involved in the acquisition and progression of tumors" ("Kick Cancer with", n.d.).

Man's utmost potent remedy for rendering the body cancer free is presumably a fruitarian diet coupled with prolonged fasting. The processes of autophagy and ketosis are triggered by prolonged fasting and are able to substantially enhance the body's innate, divine ability to terminate cancer cells and senescent cells. Moreover, when the body is fully on the mend in a prolonged fasting state, it not only deprives cancer cells of access to glucose that they need to metabolize, but also may be able to starve the cancer cells to death ("Fasting, calorie restriction", 2018), effectively abating and eliminating the tumor overtime. A tumor can be thought of as an abnormal growth of cancer cells or mass of tissues that are consolidated together.

Cancer cells are simply mutated cells and the tumor internally slaughters the valetudinarian when the tumor becomes ten centimeters wide in diameter and begins to relentlessly metastasize to other organs. Moreover, cancer cells thrive, prosper, flourish, and proliferate in an acidic environment. By attaining an alkaline body from eating only fruits and vegetables characterized by high levels of alkalinity that also have a low glycemic load, you can not only promote the growth of good bacteria in your gut and render your blood pH level above 7.35, but can also perhaps completely eliminate cancer, especially when combined with starving the cancer cells from undergoing prolonged fasting on a weekly basis. Furthermore, once the body has entered the metabolic state of ketosis from fasting, the body will churn out more ketones which will aid in the decimation of the cancer cells.

By making dietary changes to bolster immune system health, the body can more efficaciously terminate cancer cells, especially when in a fasted state since the body has divine healing mechanics which enables it to eradicate cancer cells that it recognizes as abnormal cells. When the body's energy is not being profusely vectored towards undergoing the metabolic and digestive processes during a prolonged fasting period, an eminently nourished body can earmark nearly all of its energy towards fully mending itself and can far more efficaciously eliminate cancer cells. Fasting also substantially boosts stem cell production and allows the body to create more white blood cells to dispatch to annihilate more cancer cells. Beyond augmenting the body's stem cell regeneration capabilities, fasting for over seventy two hours has also even been able to completely reset the entire immune system ("Study shows that", 2018).

The benefits of attaining an alkaline body are ineffably profound and allow your body to essentially become an anticancer microcosm since cancer cells thrive and uncontrollably proliferate in an acidic environment. Having an alkaline body promotes cellular metabolism, boosts healthy cell turnover rates, elevates oxygen levels in the blood stream, and allows your body to maintain a healthier weight. Moreover, having an alkaline body will render the individual more energetic and effervescence, will allow them to have clearer and more luscious skin, and will provide them with a more streamlined digestive system (Flynn, n.d.) Furthermore, the health benefits of have an alkaline body also encompass being able to bolster mental acuity, being able to enhance mental clarity, and being able to optimize your overall health. Additionally, attaining an alkaline body from consuming an anti-inflammatory diet as a raw fruitarian will allow the individual to stave off inflammation and substantially reduce risks for succumbing to maladies and life threatening, deadly chronic diseases.

Beyond embracing a nutrient dense, raw fruitarian diet and undergoing prolonged fasting, the process of reversing cancer can likely be further expedited by exercising daily, minimizing time allocated towards sedentariness, partaking in stress alleviating activities daily, and minimizing exposure to second hand smoke and other deleterious compounds comprised of noxious substances, such as carcinogens, neurotoxins, pathogens, and endocrine distributors. Some of the ample nutrient dense, fruits and vegetables that can potentially help reverse cancer encompass garlic, onions, leafy green vegetables, carboniferous vegetables, red grapes, and tomatoes (Metcalf, n.d.). For instance, "research shows that garlic is a cancer-fighting food. Several large studies have found that those who eat more garlic are less likely to develop various kinds of cancer, especially in digestive organs such as the esophagus, stomach, and colon. Ingredients in the pungent bulbs may keep cancer-causing substances in your body from working, or they may keep cancer cells from multiplying" (Metcalf, n.d.). Moreover, "the cruciferous vegetables, the group containing broccoli, cabbage, and cauliflower, may be particularly helpful cancer-fighting foods. Researchers have found that components in these veggies can protect you from the free radicals that damage your cells' DNA. They may also shield you from carcinogens, help slow the growth of tumors, and encourage cancer cells to die. They are also tasty and healthy addition to your anti-cancer diet" (Metcalf, n.d.). It is ultimately pivotal to make prudent dietary choices and decisions conducive to optimizing your health since the ramifications of neglecting to reverse cancer can be lethal.

Even though preventing or reversing and curing deadly chronic diseases may simply lie in embracing a raw fruitarian diet coupled with prolonged fasting, it is highly unlikely that this panacea will ever become mainstream and prevalent. The crux of the issue simply lies in the average person not having the self-discipline, drive, and tenacity to sustain embracing the fruitarian dietary regimen and periodically undergo prolonged fasting as needed to bolster their health. A nutrient dense, anti-inflammatory, antioxidant rich, anticancer, heart healthy, alkaline, raw fruitarian diet that has the potential to reverse chronic maladies, such as cancer, heart disease, and type 2 diabetes, is only limited to fruits and vegetables as food options.

Whole grains, refine grains, nuts, legumes, oils, seeds, animal carcasses, animal secretions, and synthetic products are not apart of the nutrient dense, alkaline, raw fruitarian diet. It is ill-advised to consume whole grains, refined grains, legumes, nuts, and seeds primarily because they are eminently taxing on the digestive system and are laced with anti-nutrients. Moreover, it is unwise to devour animal carcasses, animal secretions, synthetic products, oils, refined grains, whole grains, seeds, legumes, and oxidized products if the individual is looking to optimize their health, minimize inflammation, prolong their life, and mitigate as many health risks as possible. Animal products from animal carcasses and animal secretions can be highly inflammatory. Furthermore, these non-alkaline, carcinogenic, acidic, pathogenic, cholesterol laced animal products should never be consumed since they ravage the DNA and ultimately shorten the telomeres. Oils are highly oxidized and synthetic, man made products can easily be carcinogenic, pathogenic, and devoid of any essential nutrients from plant based sources which is why they should also never be consumed.

Abstaining from consuming foods outside the only two healthy food groups of fruits and vegetables is a lifestyle change that even the average ailing people is reticent to concede to embracing since they cannot envision a life devoid of their favorite animal products. The grim reality is that the tastes they may deem to be palatable from inflammatory, non-alkaline, carcinogenic, disease promoting foods, may not only be costing them decades off their lives, but also may be severely comprising their health. The average person is acutely unaware just how lethal the consumption of animal products can be towards their overall health and longevity.

Nutrient dense fruits not only essentially always taste scrumptious and succulent, but also have robust flavor profiles ranging from zesty to savory. Fruits and vegetables are sensational to the taste buds and do not need any synthetic food additives to have delectable flavor profiles.

If ailing people were not recalcitrant about making dietary changes for the prospect of potentially reversing their chronic maladies and salvaging their health instead of imprudently opting to further exacerbate their already comprised health by consuming more inflammatory, non-alkaline, carcinogenic, disease promoting foods, then they would soon learn to cope with the dietary changes as their taste buds adjust to their new fruitarian dietary regimen and would likely begin to eminently relish the robust natural flavors derived from nature's exorbitant variety of medicinal foods, fruits and vegetables. Parting with the tastes of unhealthy foods is not something the average person would ever likely advertently opt to do in spite of how deleterious their dietary decisions can be on the future states of their health. A nutrient dense, anti-inflammatory, antioxidant rich, anticancer, heart healthy, alkaline, raw fruitarian simply requires dietary trade offs that most people, even ailing people, are unwilling to make in spite of the current states of their health.

Fasting takes tremendous self discipline, time, and commitment. In spite of the ample health benefits it can confer to an individual with a healthy BMI and eminently nourished body, it is highly unlikely that the average individual will have the self discipline to abstain from eating food for a prolonged period of time, 16-72 hours. The processes of autophagy and ketosis are triggered by prolonged fasting and are able to substantially enhance the body's innate, divine ability to terminate cancer cells and senescent cells. Moreover, when the body is fully on the mend in a prolonged fasting state, it not only deprives cancer cells of access to glucose that they need to metabolize, but also may be able to starve the cancer cells to death ("Fasting, calorie restriction", 2018), effectively abating and eliminating the tumor overtime. Fasting also substantially boosts stem cell production and allows the body to create more white blood cells to dispatch to annihilate more cancer cells. Beyond augmenting the body's stem cell regeneration capabilities, fasting for over seventy two hours has also even been able to completely reset the entire immune system ("Study shows that", 2018). Not even the average ailing individual has the self discipline necessary to desist from eating food for a prolonged time window even though the health benefits can be substantial.

Moreover, the panacea to preventing, reversing, and even curing life threatening chronic diseases is unlikely to ever become mainstream since there would be far less revenue to be earned in various major industries if people were healthy, periodically fasted, and only consumed fruits and vegetables. Major industries, such as the dairy industry, meat industry, pharmaceutical industry, and candy industry, would become far less profitable if there were a major dietary shift among the population. These industries are presumably disinclined to promote the ground breaking research findings that the beneficial effects a plant based diet and fasting can have on reversing disease since it could potentially impinge on their profitability.

A pill for an ill may possibly provide systematic relief, but it does not stop the root cause of the disease. It is unlikely that any man made medication will ever allow someone to reverse and cure a disease who is unwilling to change their unhealthy dietary choices and insalubrious lifestyle habits. While a pill may possibly provide systematic relief, the average person does not understand that it does not stop the root cause of the disease. On the other hand, nature's medicine, fruits and vegetables, have the power to potentially reverse diseases, especially when coupled with the power of prolonged fasting. This natural panacea will likely never become widely promoted nor mainstream because people want to have their cake and devour it to, metaphorically speaking. In other words, you cannot expect to be cured of a chronic disease by taking a made made pill while continuing to consume unhealthy foods that are cultivating the growth of the disease and also creating an insalubrious and acidic microcosm in your body. It would also require an unprecedented level of innovation on the ends of various industries to remain profitable that presently thrive off peoples' unhealthy dietary habits if there were a paradigm shift on how people dieted and lived their lives. In spite of its potential to prevent, reverse, and even cure chronic diseases, it is unlikely that embracing a raw fruitarian diet and undergoing prolonged fasting will ever become mainstream. The average ailing person simply cannot cope with parting with the tastes of animal products or synthetic products which is truly unfortunate since the ramification of unhealthy dietary decisions can potentially be eminently devastating to their overall health and longevity. The body is only so resilient against constant stressors and needs to be properly nourished to function optimally.

Mitigating risks for life deadly chronic diseases involves following a nutrient dense, anticancer, anti-inflammatory, antioxidant rich, wholesome, heart healthy, anticancer, wholesome, alkaline, raw fruitarian diet comprised of alkaline fruits and vegetables and undergoing prolonged fasting to further optimize the health of the eminently nourished body. Embracing a nutrient dense, anti-inflammatory, antioxidant rich, raw fruitarian diet can help preempt cancer, cardiovascular disease, type 2 diabetes, kidney stones, stroke, Alzheimer's disease, and dementia. In addition to the heart healthy, nutrient dense, anticancer, anti-inflammatory, antioxidant rich, alkaline, raw fruitarian diet being able to substantially reduce the risk of succumbing to a myriad of adverse chronic diseases, it also helps preclude succumbing to inflammation and ailments and is conducive to attaining a heart healthy and brain healthy lifestyle. Dietary choices will ultimately have tremendous bearing on the future state of your health, far more so than other lifestyle factors. The benefits of making prudent dietary choices to influence your future health are often overlooked and grossly undervalued. It is ultimately deemed unwise to ever needlessly consume anything not conducive to providing you with optimal health. Making abysmal dietary decisions can bear severe repercussions on the state of your future health which is why neglectfully eating anything unhealthy you crave the taste of is deemed unwise if you ultimately desire to eminently mitigate the risks of succumbing to a deadly chronic disease.

Curing heart disease simply lies in embracing a raw fruitarian diet coupled with prolonged fasting. By eating fruits and vegetables that are characterized by high levels of alkalinity that also have a low glycemic load, such as avocados and cauliflower, you not only attain an alkaline body with a blood pH level above 7.35, but can also create a microcosm in your body that also preempts the formation of tumors and fatty plaque build up in the arteries, especially when combined with the power of prolonged fasting. "A 2014 study lead by Dr. Caldwell Esselstyn,

Jr. showed that 99.4% of 198 participants diagnosed with cardiovascular disease avoided major cardiac events when consuming a plant-based diet. Moreover, another Complete Health Improvement Program (CHIP) study that took place over six years and found that a whole food, plant-based diet, could lead to rapid reductions in chronic disease risk factors. The study recorded that a 30 day whole food, plant-based diet resulted in a significant reduction of BMI, systolic and diastolic blood pressure, cholesterol, lipoprotein cholesterol, and triglycerides for participants. Furthermore, a 2008 study reported that a plant-based diet reduced blood pressure and benefited cardiovascular disease risk by reducing serum lipids and blood pressure" ("Whole Foods Plants", n.d.). A nutrient dense, antioxidant rich, anti-inflammatory, raw fruitarian diet comprised of alkaline fruits and vegetable can also help reduce inflammation, lower cholesterol, cleanse the blood vessels of deleterious fatty deposits, and can potentially even reverse atherosclerosis by removing plaque from the artery walls. "Pioneering studies by Dr. Dean Ornish, Dr. Caldwell Esselstyn Jr., and others have shown that a plant-based diet, combined with regular exercise and a healthy overall lifestyle, can prevent, delay, and even reverse heart disease and other cardiovascular events" ("Groundbreaking research shows", n.d.).

Fasting can also be highly beneficial for reversing heart disease. Fasting has not only been discovered to reduce ample "cardiac risk factors, such as triglycerides, weight, and blood sugar levels" ("Study finds routine", 2011) , but can also help to detoxify the body. Fasting can also help reduce blood pressure, insulin resistance, inflammation, and blood cholesterol levels among providing other salubrious benefits. For instance, "studies show that fasting can increase levels of human growth hormone (HGH), an important protein hormone that plays a role in growth, metabolism, weight loss and muscle strength. Research has found that incorporating fasting into your routine may be especially beneficial when it comes to heart health" ("8 Health Benefits", 2018). Beyond embracing a nutrient dense, raw fruitarian diet and undergoing prolonged fasting, the process of reversing heart disease can likely be further expedited by pursuing heart healthy exercises daily, minimizing time allocated towards sedentariness, partaking in stress alleviating activities daily, and minimizing exposure to second hand smoke and other noxious compounds. It is ultimately pivotal to make prudent dietary choices and decisions conducive to optimizing cardiovascular health since the ramifications of neglecting to prioritize cardiovascular health can be lethal. Therefore, it is of utmost importance to undergo the requisite measures to prevent or reverse heart disease since succumbing to heart attacks, strokes, congestive heart failure, arrhythmia, plaque build up, and heart value problems can bear calamitous outcomes.

Optimizing cardiovascular health goes beyond following a heart healthy, nutrient dense, antioxidant rich, anti-inflammatory, raw fruitarian diet comprised of alkaline fruits and vegetables and undergoing prolonged fasting. It also entails pursuing heart healthy exercises daily, minimizing time earmarked towards sedentariness, partaking in stress alleviating activities daily, and minimizing exposure to second hand smoke and other hazardous compounds. By only eating alkaline fruits and vegetable and by abstaining from consuming any inflammatory foods tainted with cholesterol, such as animal carcasses and animal secretions, you can preempt ever succumbing to heart disease. Plaque can build up in the blood stream when cholesterol amalgamates with animal fats, calcium from animal products, and other noxious substances, such as trans fats (Garippo, 2017). Moreover, embracing an anti-inflammatory, raw fruitarian diet will not only help you optimize your cardiovascular health, but will also prevent your arteries walls from stiffing and accumulating plaque.

Some of the ample heart healthy foods encompass tomatoes, avocados, and leafy green vegetables (Link, 2018). "Leafy green vegetables are high in vitamin K and can help reduce blood pressure and improve arterial function. Studies show that a higher intake of leafy greens is associated with a lower risk of heart disease. Avocados are high in monounsaturated fats and potassium. They may help lower your cholesterol, blood pressure, and reduce risk of metabolic syndrome. Tomatoes are rich in lycopene and have been associated with a lower risk of heart disease and stroke" (Link, 2018). Ultimately, it is incumbent to always make prudent dietary choices and other decisions conducive to optimizing cardiovascular health since the repercussions of comprising your cardiovascular health can be fatal. The cardiovascular system cannot function optimally with diseased vessels, blood clots, structural problems, and other health issues which is why it is imperative to not overlook the importance of optimizing your cardiovascular health.

A robustly healthy, nutrient dense, antioxidant rich, anti-inflammatory, raw fruitarian diet comprised of alkaline fruits and vegetables can not only improve insulin sensitivity, reduce blood pressure, decrease HbA1c levels, help regulate blood sugar levels, and promote weight loss (A plant-based, n.d.), but also can cure type 2 diabetes, especially when combined with the power of prolonged fasting. "In a 2003 study, it was determined that a plant-based diet controlled blood sugar three times more effectively than a traditional diabetes diet that limited calories and carbohydrates. 'A plant-based diet is clearly a powerful tool for preventing, managing, and even reversing type 2 diabetes' "(A plant-based, n.d.). Moreover, fasting cannot only immensely benefit diabetics, but can also play a critical role in reversing diabetes. Fasting not only decreases blood pressure, improves insulin sensitivity, reduces blood glucose level, and provides other health benefits (Townley, 2018), but was also discovered to "significantly reverse or eliminate the need for diabetic medication" (Townley, 2018). Beyond embracing a raw fruitarian diet and undergoing prolonged fasting, exercising daily, attaining ample REM sleep, minimize time being sedentary, and partaking in stress alleviating activities can also help to more expeditiously reverse Type 2 diabetes.

Optimizing vascular health goes beyond embracing a nutrient dense, alkaline, raw fruitarian diet and undergoing prolonged fasting. It also involves exercising daily, attaining ample REM sleep, minimizing time allocated towards being sedentary, maintaining a health BMI, minimizing your exposure to second hand smoke and other deleterious ingredients that permeate the air, and partaking in stress alleviating activities daily. "A research study even found that fasting-induced anti-aging molecules keep blood vessels young" (Sandoiu, 2018) which further punctuates the importance of fasting for attaining long term vascular health. Fasting can also help detoxify the body, "lower blood pressure, control diabetes, and reduce both cholesterol and weight" ("Fasting: How Does", 2017). Ultimately, it is incumbent to implement prudent dietary choices as well as other salubrious decisions that optimize your vascular health since the ramifications of neglecting to prioritize the health of the body's vital network of blood vessels, the arteries, veins, and capillaries, can be eminently dire.

"Plant-based foods rich in antioxidants and fibre have a beneficial effect on lung health and can prevent chronic obstructive pulmonary disease (COPD). Additionally, good lung function can be linked to high intakes of vitamin C, vitamin E, beta carotene, citrus fruits, and apples" ("Chronic Lung Diseases", n.d.).

Moreover, bronchitis, asthma, and emphysema are also preventable with the consumption of an anti-inflammatory, antioxidant rich, raw fruitarian diet coupled with prolonged fasting. These nutrient dense, alkaline foods help prevent inflammation, phlegm, chest infections, airflow obstruction of the airflow passages, and breathing difficulties. Furthermore, lung disease can be averted with minimizing exposure to noxious pollutants, deleterious chemical fumes, dust, second-hand smoke (Nichols, 2017), carcinogens, neurotoxins, endocrine disruptors, irritants, and other hazardous ingredients that permeate the air. Fasting helps stave off lung disease since it allows the body to break down potentially harmful fat deposits and discharge toxins. Additionally, fasting bolsters immune system health, stimulates growth hormone production, increases white blood cell production, boosts stem cell production, and also allows the body to remove damaged cells. Fasting detoxifies the body (Maucere, 2018) and is critical for staving off lung disease.

Optimizing lung health goes beyond embracing an anti-inflammatory, antioxidant rich, raw fruitarian diet and undergoing prolonged fasting. Bolstering lung health entails slowly breathing through the nose and never through the mouth, remaining eminently hydrated at all times, attaining substantial REM sleep daily, pursuing lung healthy exercises to remain active, partaking in stress alleviating activities daily, utilizing optimal breathing techniques daily to improve oxygen inhalation, minimizing time spent being sedentary, and minimizing exposure to deleterious ingredients such as pollutants, second hand smoke, chemical fumes, dust, carcinogens, neurotoxins, endocrine disruptors and irritants that can permeate the air.

Moreover," 'laughing is a great exercise to work the abdominal muscles and increase lung capacity. It also clears out your lungs by forcing enough stale air out that it allows fresh air to enter into more areas of the lung' "("Tips for Keeping", n.d.). Additionally, eating nutrient dense, anti-inflammatory, raw, alkaline fruits and vegetables rich in antioxidants, vitamins, minerals, phytonutrients, fibre, and other salubrious compounds can significantly augment lung health ("Chronic Lung Diseases", n.d.). Some of the myriad of wholesome, nutrient dense foods that enhance lung health encompass broccoli, garlic, apples, papayas, oranges, cabbage, cauliflower, grapefruit, carrots, and red bell peppers ("14 Foods for", 2018).

Optimizing lung health is ultimately vital and of utmost importance since the lungs are necessary for extracting oxygen from the environment and subsequently transferring the oxygen into the bloodstream. The ramifications appertaining to neglecting to optimize lung health can be dire and can lead to inflammatory lung diseases, wheezing, phlegm, chest infections, and other undesirable health issues. It is incumbent to only make optimal dietary choices and prudent decisions that are conducive to optimizing lung health in order to preempt dire lung health issues and be able to breath seamlessly without succumbing to wheezing or other breathing difficulties.

Kidney disease can be offset by high blood pressure, diabetes, autoimmune diseases, blood flow issues, urinary tract problems, and other health issues ("Kidney Failure ESRD", n.d.). Embracing an anti-inflammatory, raw fruitarian diet can help lower blood pressure, prevent type 2 diabetes and autoimmune diseases, improve blood circulation, and preempt urinary tract problems. Moreover, nutrient dense, alkaline fruits and vegetables keep the body eminently hydrated since they are primarily comprised of water and help optimize kidney health.

Furthermore, the consumption of nutrient dense, alkaline fruits and vegetables devoid of oxalates and phosphates will preempt the formation of kidney stones. Ensuring that you have adequate calcium from alkaline fruits and vegetables and remain eminently hydrated will also help preclude the formation of kidney stones. Additionally, fasting bolsters kidney health while also providing a reduction of oxidative stress and blood pressure (Gunnars, 2016). Chronic kidney disease, acute kidney failure, and kidney stones can be preventable by implementing optimal dietary decisions that benefit the kidneys rather than harm the kidneys.

Optimizing kidney health goes beyond being adherent to consuming a nutrient dense, alkaline fruitarian diet comprised of anti-inflammatory fruits and vegetables that are essentially devoid of oxalates and phosphates. In order to bolster kidney health, it is imperative to attain ample REM sleep, stay hydrated at all times by drinking a copious amount of distilled water, exercise daily, pursue stress alleviating activities daily, and minimize time spent remaining sedentary by living a physically active lifestyle in order to improve blood flow, enhance glucose metabolism, and lower blood pressure. Fasting can also be pivotal for optimizing kidney health since it can help detoxify the kidneys, shed off excess weight, and reduce blood pressure. "Fasting can also boost the immune system, stimulate cellular autophagy, improve genetic repair mechanisms, improve insulin sensitivity, and reduce the risk of chronic diseases, including kidney disease. Fasting eliminates input of additional toxins and helps the body open its drainage pathways" (Nohr, n.d.).

It is ultimately crucial to optimize hydration and consume kidney healthy foods to optimize kidney health. Distilled "water supports many of your body's functions by improving oxygen delivery to cells, transporting nutrients, flushing toxins, and supporting natural healing processes" (Nohr, n.d.). Some of the many kidney health foods encompass lemons, limes, cucumbers, and celery (Nohr, n.d.). Implementing the necessary measures to optimize long term kidney health should not be overlooked since the kidneys are vital organs that are needed to filter blood and eliminate waste.

Inflammation, high blood pressure, hardening of the arteries, and animal fats can cause stroke. Succumbing to inflammation, clogged arteries, high blood pressure and even stroke, can be averted by following a nutrient dense, raw fruitarian diet. Nutrient dense, raw fruits and vegetables are devoid of cholesterol and animal fats which clog the arteries. Moreover, nutrient dense, alkaline fruits and vegetable are anti-inflammatory foods that help lower blood pressure in addition to promoting smooth, unclogged, and cleansed arteries. Additionally, fasting has been found to help substantially reduce the risk of stroke and other neurological disorders (Kandola, 2018). Preempting stroke involves adhering to an anti-inflammatory, raw fruitarian diet comprised of ample alkaline fruits and vegetables ("The Best and", n.d.) coupled with embracing prolonged fasting to render your body a stroke free microcosm.

Optimizing artery health simply involves embracing an anti-inflammatory, raw fruitarian diet and undergoing prolonged fasting. By eating only nutrient dense, anti-inflammatory, raw fruits and vegetable, you will be able to preclude blood clot obstructions and blood vessel ruptures that can be caused from implementing imprudent dietary choices. Additionally, streamlining blood flow and bolstering artery health goes beyond following an anti-inflammatory, raw fruitarian diet and undergoing prolonged fasting to help cleanse the arteries. It also entails exercising daily, attaining considerable REM sleep, and pursue stress alleviating activities daily to minimize stress. Alleviating stress is vital since the ramifications of succumbing to chronic stress can possibly culminate in increasing your blood pressure level, narrowing the blood vessels, and can potentially ravage the DNA overtime (Lu, 2014). Being sedentary and indolent is also ill-advised if you yearn to optimize your artery health, especially since sedentariness can contribute to poorer blood circulation, the formation of blood clots, inflammation, and induce other undesirable health issues. While dietary decisions, may be the greatest determinant of the future state of your health, you should not forgo making improvements to other facets of your life if ultimately desire to optimize your artery health. The long term benefits of REM sleep, exercising daily, pursue stress alleviating activities daily, and undergoing prolonged fasting are eminently profound and should not be overlooked.

Alzheimer's disease, a chronic neurodegenerative disease that causes dementia and severe cognitive decline, can be rendered preventable through making lifestyle changes that entail embracing a nutrient dense, raw fruitarian diet in tandem with prolonged fasting to optimize cognitive health.

Fasting has been found to bolster cognitive function, cognitive alertness, cognitive learning, and cognitive memory (Wnuk, 2018). "Fasting also profusely stimulates the production of the brain-derived neurotrophic factor, or BDNF. This aforementioned protein plays critical roles in learning, memory, and the generation of new nerve cells in the hippocampus. Furthermore, fasting also renders the neurons more stress resistant and also helps optimize neuroplasticity, learning, memory, and the resistance of the brain to stressors" (Wnuk, 2018).

Moreover, the consumption of nutrient dense, fruits and vegetables will help stave off Alzheimer's disease and dementia since these food groups inundated with brain healthy ingredients, such as antioxidants, vitamins, minerals, and phytonutrients that help protect the neurological system. Furthermore, the consumption of nutrient dense, alkaline fruits and vegetables not only bolster brain health and mental acuity, but also enhances memory, problem solving skills, and concentration (Webber, n.d.). Dietary choices have tremendous bearing on the individual's future cognitive health. We can either promote optimal cognitive health by creating an internal environment which the brain can flourish and repair itself or elicit a microcosm that promotes cognitive decline simply through dietary decisions. Poor nutritional choices will ravage the brain overtime (Sherzai & Sherzai, 2017) while prudent nutritional choices will nourish the brain and augment cognitive health.

Moreover, to further reduce risk of developing Alzheimer's disease and dementia, you can consume nutrient dense fruits and vegetables that contain folate. Folate not only plays a vital role in allow the body to generate new cells, but also "reduces homocysteine levels. High homocysteine levels put you at risk for both heart disease and memory loss" ("Pillar 1: Diet," n.d.). "High intakes of folate may also protect against certain cancers, including those of the breast, gut, lung and pancreas" (Julson,

2018). Folate, a type of water soluble B vitamin, can be found in citrus fruits and even leafy green vegetables, such as kale and arugula.

"Some researchers have even argued that Alzheimer's is essentially a garbage disposal problem, the brain's inability to cope with what we feed it over a lifetime. Poor nutrition damages the brain in so many ways: it causes inflammation and the buildup of oxidative by-products, clogs blood vessels, and deprives your brain of the nutrients it needs to strengthen neurons, their connections, and critical support structures" (Sherzai & Sherzai, 2017). Nutrient dense fruits and vegetables coupled with prolonged fasting are perhaps the utmost potent natural panaceas for preventing Alzheimer's disease and dementia.

Moreover, optimizing cognitive health goes beyond eating an exorbitant amount of anti-inflammatory, nutrient dense, raw fruit and vegetables and undergoing prolonged fasting. Optimizing cognitive health also entails having an active lifestyle in which you participate in physical exercises daily, pursue stress alleviating activities and mindful breathing exercises daily, maintain healthy relationships with friends and family members, attain considerable undisturbed REM sleep, and partake in multimodal activities in order to challenge and engage (Sherzai & Sherzai, 2017) multiple regions of the brain.

By only eating alkaline fruits and vegetable and by abstaining from consuming any inflammatory foods tainted with cholesterol, such as animal carcasses and animal secretions, you can preclude ever succumbing to heart disease. Plaque can build up in the blood stream when cholesterol amalgamates with animal fats, calcium from animal products, and other noxious substances, such as trans fats (Garippo, 2017). Moreover, an anti-inflammatory, raw fruitarian diet will not only optimize cardiovascular health, but will also prevent your arteries walls from stiffing and accumulating plaque. To further augment cardiovascular health, exercise and stress-relieving activities should be pursued daily since they are conducive to embracing a health life style. Furthermore, an anti-inflammatory, raw fruitarian diet coupled with prolonged fasting even has the potential to completely reverse cardiovascular disease.

Veganism has gained significant traction over the years and is falsely touted as the optimal diet which is an erroneous fallacy. Raw fruitarianism is in fact the utmost healthiest diet since it only limits food choices to the only two healthy food groups, fruits and vegetables. While veganism does promote the consumption of some health food groups, such as fruits and vegetables, it also permits the consumption of unhealthy food groups, such as whole grains and legumes. It is of vital importance to desist from consuming whole grains, refined grains, legumes, nuts, and seeds if you desire to optimize your health and avert succumbing to dire health issues, such as comprising your gut health.

Prolonged fasting combined with a raw fruitarian diet is perhaps man's greatest panacea to mitigate the ravages of time, safeguard the telomeres, and optimize health. As frugivores, the raw fruitarian diet is man's optimal diet that confers unprecedented health benefits to the individual. The raw fruitarian diet is a subset of the raw vegan diet that prioritizes the consumption of fruits for the main calorie source, whereas veganism places a greater emphasis on having a more diverse diet of any whole plant based products, such as carbohydrate dense vegetables, seeds, nuts, and whole grains. Similarity to a vegan diet, the fruitarian diet consist of eating primarily fruits and vegetables. Moreover, to optimize food choices, it is incumbent to eat only fruits and vegetables that are characterized by high levels of alkalinity and that have a low glycemic load, such as avocados, olives, coconuts, zucchini, and cauliflower, which also leave an alkaline residue in the body post being digested.

The salubrious benefits of the raw fruitarian diet are eminently profound and plentiful. Some of the ample health benefits of following the raw fruitarian diet encompass being able to be eminently hydrated since fruits are comprised of mostly 70-99% water, being able to mitigate free radical damage from having consumed the wealth of antioxidants in fruits, being able to attenuate inflammation since fruits innately have numerous anti-inflammatory properties, and being able to profusely revitalize the organs and nourish the body. Nutrient dense fruits are not only replete with phytonutrients, macronutrients, micronutrients, antioxidants, vitamins, minerals, fiber, and other salubrious compounds, but also unequivocally are the elixirs of a healthy life.

Furthermore, following the fruitarian diet will allow you to bolster cognitive functions, augment respiratory system health, enhance cardiovascular system health, and improve endocrine system and digestive system health. It will also help you detoxify the body, loose excess body fat, attain a more stable mood and substantially higher energy levels, have clearer and more vibrant skin, age more gracefully, attain keener senses, minimize digestive distress amid meals, and improve nervous system health. Moreover, adhering to the raw fruitarian diet also amplifies your sensual feelings, improves muscular coordination, averts constipation, minimizes depressive cycles, optimizes both physical health and mental health, and substantially reduce risks for deadly chronic diseases. Following a nutrient dense, raw fruitarian diet can help you curtail hunger cravings and help you optimize your physical, mental, and spiritual well being as a frugivore consuming their natural diet.

The power of the raw fruitarian diet goes beyond simply offering profound health benefits to individuals. It also simplifies meal preparations since the only work involved with preparing a raw fruitarian meal involves washing off the raw fruit before consumption. There is no cooking involved in the process and the skins and peels of a preponderance of fruits, such as mangoes, kiwis, and grapefruits, can be consumed, contrary to what many people have erroneously disbelieved. Additionally, raw fruitarian meals are always scrumptious, delectable, and palatable since fruits are nutrient dense and have robust flavor profiles. Therefore, eating a meal as a raw fruitarian becomes a euphoric and sensational experience that will not only help you to detoxify your vessel (Fruitarianism, 2018), but will also imbue you with indefatigable energy and allow you to function at a higher vibrational frequency. The fruitarian diet is able to promote optimal physical, mental, and spiritual health. Moreover, a raw, nutrient dense fruitarian diet also can not only help prevent you from succumbing to inflammation, ailing, and chronic diseases, but can also possibly help reverse deadly chronic diseases, such as type two diabetes, especially when coupled with prolonged fasting.

Moreover, individuals should not only consume fruits and vegetable in their raw, natural forms, but should also only drink distilled water devoid of the acute neurotoxin, sodium fluoride, and other noxious ingredients, such as chlorine, trihalomethanes, and nitrates, that taint the tap water supply. By utilizing a quality water purification system that renders water distilled, such as the Propur water filter, you can drink purified, non-tainted water. It is also ill-advised to ever consume anything oxidized, such as extra virgin oils or smoothies.

Robustly healthy, nutrient dense fruits and vegetables should be profusely eaten amid meals and should be eaten in a specific order to minimize digestive distress. Moreover, vegan supplements for obtaining nutrients and vitamins your diet may be devoid of should be consumed at least fifteen minutes before devouring a meal. In order to optimize food combing you may want to eat foods in the following order: acidic fruits first, sub-acidic fruits second, sweet fruits third, protein dense vegetables fourth, carbohydrate dense vegetables fifth, and fat dense fruits fruits last. Frozen fruits and vegetables foods are the utmost nutrient dense foods as a result of not having succumbed to the ravages of oxidation which allows them to retain the majority of their nutrients. Furthermore, fruits and vegetables should ideally always be eaten raw so that their enzymes, nutrients, vitamins, and minerals are not decimated before consumption. Cooking fruits and vegetables can mutilate the foods and comprises their innate nutrient profiles.

Moreover, as previously punctuated, it is always imperative that you consume vegan supplements from plant based sources of nutrients and vitamins that your diet may be devoid of, such as Vitamin B12, Nascent Iodine, and Vitamin D3, to ensure that your body has all the requisite nutrients it needs to attain robust, vigorous health. By eating only fruits and vegetables that have low glycemic loads and that are characterized by high levels of alkalinity, meaning they leave an alkaline residue of 7.0 or above post being digested, you can attain an alkaline body and perhaps even circumvent the formation tumors since cancer cells needs an acidic environment to survive, prosper, and proliferate. The only part of the vessel that should be highly acidic is the stomach with a PH level of 6 or below to disintegrate anything that enters into it so that you vessel does not become a repository for waste and store food products for prolonged periods of time in the form of belly fat.

It is always incumbent to get your blood tested to ensure that your vessel has all the nutrients it needs for optimal health at all times. You can refine your diet as need by incorporating a wider variety of nutrient dense fruits and vegetables into your diet if your blood tests indicate your vessel is lacking a nutrient, such as non-heme iron. By having access to the blood test results, you can make dietary changes, such as by profusely eating olives in this example to rectify an iron deficiency you might be succumbing to encountering.

As previously mentioned, before you undergo a prolonged fast, you want to ensure that you have a healthy BMI of well above 18.5, have recently consumed a copious amount of nutrient dense fruits and vegetables to nourish the vessel, are eminently hydrated, and do not have to do anything too physical intense amid this fasting period. I personally attempt to eat 5,000-20,000 calories per meal before undergoing a prolonged fast.

Amid the prolonged fasting period, you can enter ketosis within a 24 hour period by dry fasting or alternatively enter ketosis within a 72 hour period by water fasting. If you opt to dry fast only for the initial 24 hours of the prolonged fast, you can enter ketosis in one third the time then you otherwise would if you were going to water fast through the entirety of the prolonged fast. It is always advised to be eminently hydrated and never dehydrated. Furthermore, if you opt to dry fast for the initial 24 hours amid the prolonged fast then you should always drink distilled water after the 24 hour period has elapsed. I personally do not go for any longer than 24 hours without distilled water.

Once you have entered ketosis during the prolonged fast, your body can be fully on the mend since no energy is diverted away from the healing process. When your vessel is undergoing a prolonged fast, it is fully in healing mode, and you are able to exploit the body's divine healing mechanisms to terminate far more cancer cells and senescent cells than you otherwise would when not fasting. During a prolonged fast, energy is not be diverted towards the digestive system processes since no calories are entering the bloodstream.

Moreover, the benefits of undergoing autophagy and ketosis are eminently salubrious. During a prolonged fast, the HDL cholesterol levels will increase, blood pressure levels will decrease, insulin sensitivity will be bolstered, cardiovascular health will be improved, and your immune system health will be augmented. Additionally many other health benefits can be reaped during a prolonged fast such as the amplification of growth hormone production, increased stem cell production, the suppression of inflammation, the normalization of ghrelin levels, the plummeting of triglyceride levels, and the bolstering of cognitive function. Furthermore, prolonged fasting will allow your cells to become more resilient and you will also boost telomere activity. Additionally, you will better be able to mitigate your risks of succumbing to chronic diseases (Link, 2018) as your vessel is able to detoxify itself by undergoing a prolonged fast. A prolonged fast is typically 24-96 hours in length and can be utilized as the panacea combined with a raw fruitarian diet to help you easily optimize health, maximize your longevity rate, and avert succumbing to chronic diseases.

As frugivores with long intestines, high PH levels, and flat teeth, it is incumbent that our species only devours foods from foods groups that we have the anatomy to efficaciously digest, such as fruits and vegetables. It is unwise to devour animal carcasses, animal secretions, synthetic products, oils, refined grains, whole grains, seeds, legumes, and oxidized products if the individual is looking to optimize their health, minimize inflammation, prolong their life, and substantially mitigate as many health risks as possible. We currently cannot modify our innate genetic code and should ideally resort to following a diet of only consuming fruits and vegetables that optimize our health and maximize our longevity rate.

Fruits and vegetables are replete with vitamins, minerals, carotenoids, phytonutrients, antioxidants, fiber, and other salubrious compounds that we need to be able to thrive, prosper, and flourish. The health benefits reaped and the nutrient profiles will vary per fruit or vegetable, with some foods being far healthier to consume than others.

Ultimately, reaping the benefits of prolonged fasting coupled with embracing a heart healthy, anticancer, nutrient dense, antioxidant rich, anti-inflammatory, alkaline, raw fruitarian diet can be profound and can help you easily optimize health, maximize your longevity rate, and substantially reduce risks of succumbing to deadly chronic diseases. The health benefits of prolonged fasting are often overlooked, but should not be neglected since it is perhaps the body's most potent way to exploit its divine healing mechanisms to mend itself since all of its energy is full concentrated on detoxifying the vessel during a prolonged fast. In conclusion, prolonged fasting combined with a raw fruitarian diet is perhaps man's greatest natural panacea for attaining the utmost highest form of robust, unalloyed health.

Atkins Desserts Recipes

Black Velvet Cupcakes

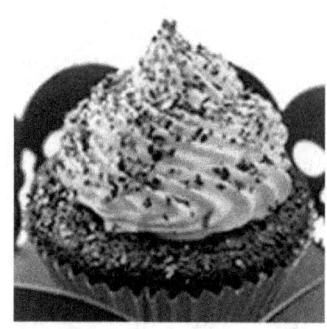

Servings: 6 | Prep: 5 m | Style: American | Cook: 17 m

Ingredients

- 3 large Eggs (Whole)
- 1/4 cup Coconut Milk Unsweetened
- 1/4 cup Xylitol
- 2 tsps Vanilla Extract
- 7 tbsps Unsalted Butter Stick
- 1/4 cup Organic High Fiber Coconut Flour
- 1/4 tsp Baking Powder (Straight Phosphate, Double Acting)
- 2 tbsps Cocoa Powder (Unsweetened)
- 1/4 tsp Baking Soda
- 1/4 tsp Salt
- 4 oz Cream Cheese
- 6 tsps Erythritol

Directions

For this recipe you will need black food coloring (either liquid or gel; for liquid you will need 1/2 tsp and for gel just a small amount is needed). You will also need orange or other color for the frosting; amount will depend upon desire for color depth. The cupcakes may be sprinkled with edible glitter which is made of food coloring and guar gum (no sugar). The glitter and food colorings can be found at some hobby stores or online.

1. Preheat oven to 375°F. Prepare a muffin tin with 6 paper cups. Set aside.
2. In a medium bowl whisk the eggs with the coconut milk, granular sugar substitute, vanilla, black food coloring and 3 tablespoons melted butter. Set aside.
3. In a small bowl whisk together the coconut flour, baking powder, cocoa powder, baking soda and salt. Add to egg mixture whisking to incorporate all ingredients for about a minute. Divide batter into the 6 paper cups, place in the oven and bake until fully set in the center; about 15-18 minutes. When done, set on a wire rack to cool.
4. Make Frosting: In a small bowl, beat the cream cheese with an electric mixer until smooth. Add 4 tbsp (1/4 cup) softened butter and continue to beat another minute. Add the erythritol; beat another minute then add vanilla and food coloring as desired. Adjust for sweetness by adding a pinch of stevia if desired. Frost cupcakes using a piping bag or by hand.

Nutritional Information
- Protein : 5.4g

- Fat : 23.3g
- Fiber : 10.3g
- Calories :269

Caramelized Pear Custard

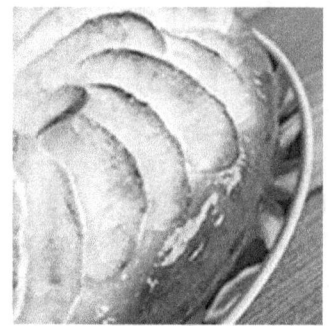

Servings: 8 | Prep: 5 m | Style: American | Cook: 20 m

Ingredients
- 2 tbsps Butter
- 2 tbsps Xylitol
- 1/4 tsp ground Cardamom
- 2 medium (approx 2-1/2 per lb) Pears
- 3 large Eggs (Whole)
- 2 large Egg Yolks
- 2 cups Heavy Cream
- 1/8 cup Sugar Free Low Calorie Maple Flavor Syrup
- 1/2 fl oz (no ice) Rum
- 1 tsp Vanilla Extract

Directions
1. Preheat oven to 375°F.

2. Heat the butter, xylitol and cardamom in a large sauce pan over medium-high heat. Slice the pears into 1/2-inch wedges. Once the butter has melted add the pears and allow to caramelized for 4 minutes on each side. Remove from heat and arrange in a pie plate or 3-4 cup casserole dish. Reserve about 2 Tbsp syrup and pour the remaining over the pears (keep remaining in the sauce pan and set aside).
3. In a small bowl, whisk the eggs, egg yolks, heavy cream, sugar free syrup, rum and vanilla until combined. Pour mixture over the pears and bake for 15-20 minutes until golden brown and custard has set. Remove from oven and allow to cool slightly.
4. Using a pastry brush, brush the top with reserved caramel syrup. If the syrup has hardened, reheat in the sauce pan until liquid.

Nutritional Information
- Protein : 4.4g
- Fat : 27.9g
- Fiber : 1.3g
- Calories :310

Cardamom Butter Cookies

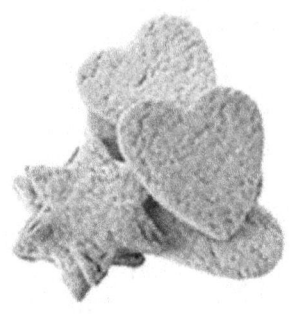

Servings: 12 | Prep: 10 m | Style: American | Cook: 23 m

Ingredients

- 1/2 cup Blanched Almond Flour
- 1/4 tsp Baking Powder (Straight Phosphate, Double Acting)
- 1/2 tsp Salt
- 10 tbsps Unsalted Butter Stick
- 1/2 cup Sucralose Based Sweetener (Sugar Substitute)
- 1 large Egg (Whole)
- 1 tbsp Tap Water
- 2 tsps Vanilla Extract
- 4 2/3 servings All Purpose Low-Carb Baking Mix
- 3/4 tsp ground Cardamom

Directions

Please use the Atkins recipe for All Purpose Low-Carb Baking Mix (or the Gluten Free version) for this recipe. To make 12 servings you will need 1 1/2 cups of the mix. If you change the serving size for the recipe to up or downsize it you will need to adjust accordingly. Each serving of bake mix is 1/3 cup.

1. Heat oven to 350°F. Line 2 baking sheets with parchment paper; set aside.
2. Combine 1 1/2 cups baking mix, 1/2 cup almond flourl, baking powder, and salt in a medium bowl. Combine butter and sugar substitute in a large bowl; cream with an electric mixer on high speed until light and fluffy. Add egg, water, vanilla, and cardamom; beat on medium speed until combined, scraping down sides of bowl as necessary (mixture may look watery). Add flour mixture; mix on low speed until dough comes together.
3. Divide dough in half, and then in half again. Make 6 equal balls from each quarter portion of dough. Place 12 balls on each baking sheet. Press each gently with the tines of a fork in a crisscross pattern (optional); bake until lightly browned on the edges, about 10 minutes. Alternatively, place in the refrigerator for 30 minutes and then roll out between parchment; cut out shapes and bake. Transfer cookies to a wire rack to cool completely. Store in an airtight container for up to 1 week. Makes 2 cookies per serving.

Nutritional Information
- Protein : 13.4g
- Fat : 14g
- Fiber : 1.7g
- Calories :196

Cherry Cobbler

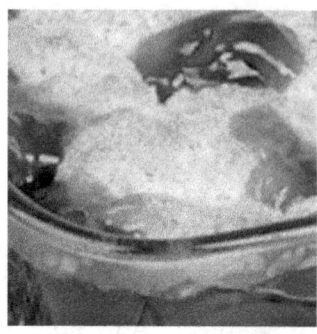

Servings: 8 | Prep: 30 m | Style: American | Cook: 40 m

Ingredients

- 1/4 cup half Pecans
- 1/2 cup Sucralose Based Sweetener (Sugar Substitute)
- 3/4 tsp Cinnamon
- 1/4 tsp Salt
- 3 tbsps Unsalted Butter Stick
- 1/3 cup Heavy Cream
- 2 tbsps Sour Cream (Cultured)
- 1 large Egg (Whole)
- 3 cup, without pits Sweet Cherries
- 1/4 tsp Pure Almond Extract
- 2 1/4 servings All Purpose Low-Carb Baking Mix

Directions

Use the Atkins recipe to make All Purpose Low-Carb Baking Mix for this recipe. You will need 3/4 cup.

1. For biscuit: In a food processor, pulse baking mix, pecans, 2 tablespoons sugar substitute, 1/2 teaspoon cinnamon and salt until medium ground. Add butter and pulse until mixture resembles a coarse meal.
2. In a liquid measuring cup or bowl, whisk heavy cream, sour cream and an egg. Pour into food processor and pulse just until combined. Remove dough and pat into a flat disk. Cover with plastic wrap and chill 1 to 2 hours.
3. For filling and cobbler: Preheat oven to 400°F. In a medium bowl, toss cherries with 1/3 cup sugar substitute, almond extract and 1/4 teaspoon cinnamon. Pour filling into an 8-inch square or round baking dish. Divide dough into 8 pieces and pat into disks about 3 across.
4. Stagger biscuits over filling and bake cobbler 35 to 40 minutes, until biscuits are browned and cooked through and fruits are bubbly and tender. Serve with freshly whipped cream (optional).

Nutritional Information
- Protein : 10.7g
- Fat : 12.9g
- Fiber : 1.3g
- Calories :191

Cherry Hazelnut Biscotti

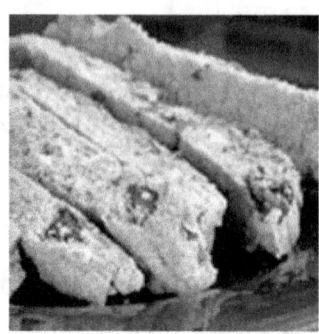

Servings: 8 | Prep: 90 m | Style: Italian | Cook: 51 m

Ingredients

- 1 1/2 cups chopped Hazelnuts or Filberts
- 1 cup Whole Grain Soy Flour
- 3/4 cup Sucralose Based Sweetener (Sugar Substitute)
- 1 tsp Cinnamon
- 1/4 cup Sour Cream (Cultured)
- 4 large Eggs (Whole)
- 12 tbsps Unsalted Butter Stick
- 1/3 cup Bake-Dried Cherries
- 1/4 tsp Salt

Directions

1. Heat oven to 350°F.
2. Whisk together finely chopped hazelnuts, soy flour, ground cinnamon and salt. In a medium bowl mix sour cream, and eggs.

3. In a large bowl, with an electric mixer on medium speed, beat butter with sugar substitute for 3 minutes until creamy.
4. Add half the egg mixture, beat 30 seconds and scrape down the sides of the bowl with spatula. Repeat with remaining egg mixture. Turn mixer on low and add dry ingredients, mixing until just combined. Fold in cherries and coarsely chopped hazelnuts. Chill dough for 1 hour.
5. Divide dough in half. On ungreased baking sheets, form each dough half into a log measuring 12 x 2½ inches (moisten hands if necessary to keep dough from sticking). Bake logs 30 minutes, until almost firm. Transfer sheets to wire rack to cool 10 minutes.
6. Reduce oven temperature to 325°F. Carefully cut logs crosswise, with a serrated knife, into ½ wide slices. Arrange slices on baking sheets. Bake 17-20 minutes until firm and crisp. Cool slices on baking sheets before storing.

Nutritional Information
- Protein : 2.1g
- Fat : 7.2g
- Fiber : 0.8g
- Calories :82

Chocolate And Flan Layered Mini Cakes

Servings: 8 | Prep: 20 m | Style: American | Cook: 50 m

Ingredients
- 2 1/2 tbsps Organic 100% Whole Ground Golden Flaxseed Meal
- 2 tsps Cocoa Powder (Unsweetened)
- 1/8 tsp Baking Soda
- 1/16 tsp Salt

- 2 large Eggs (Whole)
- 2 oz Sugar Free Chocolate Chips
- 1 1/2 tbsps Unsalted Butter Stick
- 1 tbsp Tap Water
- 2 tbsps Sour Cream (Cultured)
- 1 tsp Vanilla Extract
- 3 tbsps Cream Cheese
- 3/4 cup Heavy Cream
- 2/3 cup Coconut Cream
- 1 large Egg Yolk
- 2 tbsps Sucralose Based Sweetener (Sugar Substitute)
- 6 tbsps Sugar Free Caramel Syrup

Directions

Note: For best results, this recipe requires 6 hours of refrigeration before serving.

For the Cake:

1. Preheat oven to 350°F and adjust rack to the middle position. Grease six wells of a muffin tin.
2. Combine the flax meal, cocoa, baking soda and salt in a small bowl; set aside.
3. In a medium microwave safe bowl, combine the chocolate and butter. Microwave at 30 second intervals, stirring at each interval until melted; about 3 minutes total.
4. Whisk together the water, sour cream, 1/2 egg and 1/2 tsp vanilla. Add to the melted chocolate and stir until fully incorporated.
5. Stir in flax mixture until just combined. Divide the batter equally among the six muffin wells.

For the Flan:

1. Combine the cream cheese, heavy cream, coconut milk, 1 1/2 eggs, egg yolk, granular sugar substitute and 1/2 tsp vanilla in a blender and blend until smooth.
2. Pour the flan mixture over the cake batter until almost filled to the top. Place muffin tin in a large roasting pan and fill roasting pan with hot water until it reaches halfway up the sides of the muffin wells.
3. Bake until a toothpick inserted in the cake comes out clean and the flan reaches 180°F. As it cooks the cake will rise to the top of the muffin tin and the flan will remain below, if the cake is done on top and it has cooked for at least 50 minutes the flan should be the correct temperature.
4. Transfer the muffin tin to a wire rack and allow it to cool to room temperature, about 1 hour, cover with plastic wrap and refrigerate until fully set, about 6 hours or overnight.
5. To release the cakes, place bottom of muffin tin in the same roasting pan used for cooking and fill with 1-inch of hot tap water; allow to sit for 1 minute. Gently turn muffin tin upside down to release the flan and carefully transfer each to serving plates.
6. Drizzle 2 tablespoons sugar-free caramel or maple syrup over the cakes before serving.

Nutritional Information
- Protein : 5.1g
- Fat : 27.5g
- Fiber : 1.4g
- Calories :281

Chocolate Donut Delight

Servings: 6 | Prep: 5 m | Style: American | Cook: 13 m

Ingredients

- 1 large Egg (Whole)
- 4 oz Almond Butter
- 2 tbsps Cocoa Powder (Unsweetened)
- 6 tsps Erythritol
- 1/4 tsp Baking Powder (Straight Phosphate, Double Acting)
- 1/4 tsp Baking Soda
- 1/4 tsp Salt
- 1/2 14 oz can Coconut Cream
- 2 tsps Vanilla Extract

Directions

Note: For best results, this recipe requires 6 hours of refrigeration before serving.

For the Cake:

1. Preheat oven to 350°F and adjust rack to the middle position. Grease six wells of a muffin tin.
2. Combine the flax meal, cocoa, baking soda and salt in a small bowl; set aside.
3. In a medThis recipe is suitable for all phases except for the first two weeks of Induction due to the almond butter.
4. Preheat oven to 350°F. Prepare a 6-well donut pan with non-stick spray.
5. Place all ingredients in a blender or food processor, pulse a few times, scraping the container between pulses.
6. Pour into donut pan and bake for 13 minutes. Cool in pan for 10 minutes then turn out on a wire rack to cool completely.

Nutritional Information
- Protein : 6.2g

- Fat : 15.8g
- Fiber : 2.9g
- Calories :180

Chocolate Ice Cream

Servings: 8 | Prep: 240 m | Style: American | Cook: 10 m

Ingredients

- 2 cups Heavy Cream
- 4 large Egg Yolks
- 10 packets Sucralose Based Sweetener (Sugar Substitute)
- 1/4 cup Cocoa Powder (Unsweetened)
- 2 tbsps Sugar Free Chocolate Syrup
- 1 tsp Vanilla Extract

Directions

1. Heat cream in a heavy saucepan over low heat. Whisk in egg yolks, one at a time. Cook over low heat, stirring constantly, until mixture coats the back of a spoon. Do not let boil.
2. Remove from heat. Whisk in sugar substitute, cocoa powder, chocolate syrup, and vanilla extract.
3. Cool to room temperature. Pour custard into an ice cream maker and freeze according to manufacturers instructions.

Nutritional Information

- Protein : 3.2g
- Fat : 24.8g
- Fiber : 1g
- Calories :249

Chocolate Mint Cheesecake Bars

Servings: 24 | Prep: 270 m | Style: American | Cook: 20 m

Ingredients

- 2 oz Unsweetened Baking Chocolate Squares
- 2 1/4 cups Heavy Cream
- 1/4 cup Unsalted Butter Stick
- 1/2 cup Erythritol Powder
- 2 tsps Vanilla Extract
- 2 large Eggs (Whole)
- 1 1/3 cups Tap Water
- 1 3/4 cups Sucralose Based Sweetener (Sugar Substitute)
- 1/4 cup Cocoa Powder (Unsweetened)
- 1 cup Blanched Almond Flour
- 1 1/2 tsps Baking Powder (Straight Phosphate, Double Acting)
- 1/2 tsp Salt
- 1 package (1 oz) Gelatin Powder (Unsweetened)
- 16 oz Cream Cheese
- 1 tsp extract of Peppermint (Mint)
- 8 tbsps Sugar Free Chocolate Syrup

Directions

Be sure to use powdered erythritol (you will need about 1/2 cup granulated to make 1 cup powdered). It can be easily powdered in a blender. Measure it after it is powdered.

Bottom layer:

1. Preheat an oven to 350°F and grease a 9x13x2-inch non-stick pan; set aside. Melt the chocolate and 1/4 cup heavy cream in a small bowl in the microwave at 20 second intervals. Once melted mix to combine and set aside to cool.
2. Cream the butter and 1 cup powdered erythritol in a mixer for 5 minutes until light and fluffy. Add the vanilla and the eggs one at a time blending for 30 seconds between each egg. Add the cooled chocolate mixture, beating until thoroughly combined. Add 1/3 cup water and 1/2 cup sucralose, beat for 1 minute.
3. In a small bowl whisk together the cocoa powder, almond flour, baking powder and salt. Add to the batter and mix for another minute until fully blended. Pour batter into prepared pan and bake for 20 minutes or until a toothpick inserted in the center comes out clean. Allow to cool. While cooling prepare the top layer.

Top layer:

1. Add the packet of gelatin to 1 cup boiling water. Mix until all the gelatin dissolves then place in the refrigerator about 10 minutes (do not allow it to fully set-up, cool to room temperature only.)
2. In a medium bowl beat the softened cream cheese with 1 cup sucralose until fully blended and smooth. Add the peppermint extract and enough green food coloring to achieve desired color depth (about 1/4 teaspoon). When the gelatin has fully cooled, blend it into the cheese mixture.
3. Whip the remaining 2 cups cream with the remaining 1/4 cup sucralose until semi-stiff peaks form. Gently fold the cream into the cheese mixture until fully incorporated. Pour this over the cooled brownie layer in the pan and refrigerate for 4 hours or overnight.
4. When ready to serve, cut into 24 squares and top with 1 teaspoon of sugar-free chocolate syrup (Smucker's Sugar

Free Sundae Syrup works great as it is a little thicker than regular syrup.) To make spider web: starting in the middle of the square make a spiral. Take a toothpick and from the center pull out in a straight line to the outer edge. Repeat 5-6 times spacing them equally.

Nutritional Information

- Protein : 4g
- Fat : 20.9g
- Fiber : 1.4g
- Calories :231

Chocolate Mousse Mini Cheesecakes

Servings: 8 | Prep: 270 m | Style: American | Cook: 20 m

Ingredients

- 3 oz Unsweetened Baking Chocolate Squares
- 16 oz Cream Cheese
- 1/2 cup Sucralose Based Sweetener (Sugar Substitute)
- 3 large Eggs (Whole)
- 3/4 cup Heavy Cream
- 3/4 tsp Pure Almond Extract
- 1/2 tsp Vanilla Extract

Directions

Prep time includes 4 hours to chill. You'll need to bake the cheesecakes in a water bath. If you don't have instant boiling water, begin to boil a pot of water after Step 4. This recipe can be prepared ahead of time; wrap each custard cup tightly in plastic, place in an airtight container and freeze for up to 1 month.

1. Heat oven to 325°F.
2. Place eight 6-ounce ramekins in a roasting pan; set aside.
3. Heat chocolate in the microwave in 30-second increments until fully melted, about 1-2 minutes; set aside to cool slightly.
4. In the large bowl of an electric mixer, beat cream cheese on medium speed until lightened, scraping down sides of bowl as needed. Add chocolate and beat until combined. Add sugar substitute, beating until combined.
5. Add eggs, one at a time, beating well after each addition. Add cream and almond and vanilla extracts, beating until completely smooth.
6. Pour mixture into prepared custard cups. Carefully pour enough boiling water into roasting pan to come halfway up sides of ramekins.
7. Bake until the cheesecakes are puffed and the centers are just set, about 20 minutes. Remove from oven and let sit in the water bath for 10 minutes.
8. Transfer custard cups to a wire rack; cool to room temperature. Refrigerate until well chilled, 4 hours or overnight.
9. Garnish with mint sprigs, chocolate shavings and raspberries, if desired.

Nutritional Information
- Protein : 6.8g
- Fat : 34.8g
- Fiber : 1.5g
- Calories :359

Chocolate Mudslide

Servings: 4 | Prep: 120 m | Style: American | Cook: 10 m

Ingredients

- 1 cup Heavy Cream
- 1/2 cup Tap Water
- 8 tbsps Sugar Free Chocolate Syrup
- 3 tbsps Cocoa Powder (Unsweetened)
- 1 tsp Vanilla Extract

Directions

1. In a medium saucepan combine cream, 1/2 cup syrup, water and cocoa powder.
2. Bring to a boil over medium heat.
3. Reduce heat to low; cook, stirring occasionally, 5 minutes. Remove from heat and stir in vanilla.
4. Pour mixture into two ice cube trays. Freeze 2 hours.
5. Before serving transfer cubes into a food processor and process until mixture is finely chopped and slushy. Serve immediately.

Nutritional Information

- Protein : 3g
- Fat : 22.8g
- Fiber : 2.3g
- Calories :234

Chocolate Peanut Butter Haystacks

Servings: 18 | Prep: 10 m | Style: American | Cook: 5 m

Ingredients

- 1/4 cup Heavy Cream
- 2 tbsps Unsalted Butter Stick
- 3 tbsps Cocoa Powder (Unsweetened)
- 2 tbsps Xylitol
- 1 pinch Stevia
- 1/16 tsp Salt
- 1/4 cup Natural Creamy Peanut Butter 1/3 Less Sodium & Sugar
- 2 cups Unsweetened Flaked Coconut

Directions

1. Toast the coconut flakes on a sheet pan for 5 minutes at 350°F. Once toasted, fold into the chocolate mixture until coated.
2. Drop by tablespoons onto wax paper or a silicon mat on a sheet pan forming 18 mounds. Allow to cool and harden or place in refrigerator to harden quickly. May be stored in the refrigerator in an air tight container for up to two weeks or frozen for up to 3 months. Serve cold or at room temperature. One haystack = 1 serving.

Nutritional Information

- Protein : 1.7g
- Fat : 11g
- Fiber : 3.1g
- Calories :122

Chocolate Peppermint Cupcakes

Servings: 6 | Prep: 15 m | Style: American | Cook: 17 m

Ingredients

- 1 large Eggs (Whole)
- 1/4 cup Coconut Milk Unsweetened
- 1/4 cup Xylitol
- 1 tsp Vanilla Extract
- 7 tbsps Unsalted Butter Stick
- 4 tbsps Organic High Fiber Coconut Flour
- 2 tbsps Cocoa Powder (Unsweetened)
- 1/4 tsp Baking Powder (Straight Phosphate, Double Acting)
- 1/4 tsp Salt
- 4 oz Cream Cheese
- 6 tsps Erythritol
- 1 serving Bob's Starlight Mints Peppermint Sugar Free Candy

Directions

1. Please powder the erythritol before making the frosting for this recipe. Place 2 tablespoons in a blender and pulse 3-4 times until powdered. To crush peppermint candies place them in a zip top bag and hit with a hammer.
2. Preheat oven to 375°F. Prepare a muffin tin with 6 paper cups. Set aside.
3. In a medium bowl whisk the eggs with the coconut milk, granular sugar substitute, vanilla, peppermint extract and 3 tablespoons melted butter. Set aside.
4. In a small bowl whisk together the coconut flour, cocoa powder, baking powder and salt. Add to egg mixture whisking to incorporate all ingredients for about a minute. Pour into the 6 paper cups, place in the oven and bake until fully set in the center; about 15-18 minutes. When done, set on a wire rack to cool.
5. Make Frosting: In a small bowl, beat the cream cheese with an electric mixer until smooth. Add 1/4 cup softened butter and continue to beat another minute. Add the powdered erythritol; beat another minute then add peppermint extract

and food coloring as desired (optional; red is pretty as pictured and green is festive with the red and white candies). Adjust for sweetness by adding a pinch of stevia if desired. Frost cupcakes using a piping bag or by hand. Sprinkle with crushed peppermint candies.

Nutritional Information
- Protein : 5.4g
- Fat : 23.3g
- Fiber : 10.4g
- Calories :276

Chocolate Walnut Cookies

Servings: 32 | Prep: 20 m | Style: American | Cook: 6 m

Ingredients
- 1/8 cup 100% Stone Ground Whole Wheat Pastry Flour
- 2 tbsps Whole Grain Soy Flour
- 1/8 tsp Baking Soda
- 3/4 cup Sucralose Based Sweetener (Sugar Substitute)
- 1 1/2 oz Unsweetened Baking Chocolate Squares
- 5 tbsps Heavy Cream
- 2 large Eggs (Whole)
- 2 tbsps Unsalted Butter Stick
- 1 tsp Vanilla Extract
- 1/4 cup chopped English Walnuts

Directions
1. Preheat over to 350°F. Lightly toast walnuts in an even layer on a cookie sheet for 6 to 8 minutes. Cool, coarsely chop the walnuts and set aside.
2. Put oven up to 375°F. Line two baking sheets with parchment paper or aluminum foil; set aside.

3. Whisk 2 tbsp whole-wheat flour, 2 tbsp soy flour and baking soda together in a bowl; set aside.
4. In the large bowl of an electric mixer, beat eggs and sugar substitute together on medium until light and slightly thickened. Place chocolate, cream and butter in a microwavable bowl; microwave on medium until butter has melted and chocolate has softened (it need not be completely melted), 1½ to 2 minutes. Let stand 5 minutes; stir until smooth.
5. Gradually beat the slightly warm chocolate mixture and vanilla extract into the egg mixture. Reduce speed to low, and beat in flour mixture, just until combined. Cover, and chill until thickened, 30 minutes.
6. Drop slightly rounded teaspoonfuls of dough, 1 inch apart, onto prepared sheet. Sprinkle tops of cookies with walnuts, lightly pressing into dough. Bake until cookies are just set but soft on top, 5½ to 6 minutes. Cool cookies on baking sheet 1 minute before transferring to wire racks to cool completely. Store in an airtight container.

Nutritional Information

- Protein : 0.9g
- Fat : 3.2g
- Fiber : 0.4g
- Calories :37

Chocolate Yule Log

Servings: 10 | Prep: 20 m | Style: American | Cook: 12 m

Ingredients

- 1/3 second spray Original Canola Cooking Spray
- 1 1/3 cups Sucralose Based Sweetener (Sugar Substitute)
- 5 tbsps Cocoa Powder (Unsweetened)

- 9 large Eggs (Whole)
- 2 tbsps Whole Grain Soy Flour
- 1/4 tsp Salt
- 1 1/3 cups Heavy Cream
- 2 oz Unsweetened Baking Chocolate Squares
- 8 tbsps Unsalted Butter Stick
- 1/4 tsp Vanilla Extract

Directions

1. Preheat oven to 375°F. Spray a jellyroll pan with oil spray; line with parchment, leaving a 2-inch border, spray again. Set aside.
2. In a large bowl, whisk together 1 cup sugar substitute, 4 tablespoons cocoa powder and soy flour.
3. In another large bowl, beat egg yolks with an electric mixer on high speed until pale yellow and fluffy, about 3 minutes. Turn speed down to low and slowly mix in cocoa mixture until just combined.
4. In another bowl, beat egg whites and salt with an electric mixer on high speed until stiff peaks form, about 3 minutes. Fold 1/3 of the whites into yolk mixture until just combined. Fold in remaining egg whites. Spread batter evenly in prepared pan. Bake 15 minutes, until cake springs back when lightly touched and pulls away from sides of the pan. Cool cake in pan on wire rack for 30 minutes to 1 hour.
5. While cake is cooling, prepare filling and frosting. For the filling, whip 1 cup cream and 1 1/2 tablespoon sugar substitute in a medium bowl until stiff peaks form (do not overbeat).
6. For the frosting, gradually combine 1/3 cup cream and melted chocolate in a large bowl. With an electric mixer on medium speed, beat in butter, 5 tablespoons sugar substitute, 1 tablespoon cocoa powder and vanilla. Beat until smooth and fluffy, about 4 minutes. Chill in refrigerator until ready to use.

7. When cake is cool, slide cake from pan with parchment underneath. Place on counter top. Spread filling over cake, leaving a ½ inch border. Roll up cake from narrow end, using parchment to help. Cut 1-inch diagonal pieces from each end. Transfer roll to a serving platter; place cut diagonal pieces on either side to form log stumps. Set aside.
8. To assemble: Use a generous dab of frosting to attach stumps to main log. Frost entire log, and run fork tines through frosting to create a bark-like texture.

Nutritional Information
- Protein : 7.8g
- Fat : 28.7g
- Fiber : 1.9g
- Calories :308

Chocolate-Cappuccino Mini Cupcakes

Servings: 18 | Prep: 15 m | Style: Other | Cook: 20 m

Ingredients
- 1 cup sliced Almonds
- 1 cup Whole Grain Soy Flour
- 1 tsp Baking Powder (Straight Phosphate, Double Acting)
- 1/2 cup Unsalted Butter Stick
- 1/2 cup Sucralose Based Sweetener (Sugar Substitute)
- 1 tbsp Cocoa Powder (Unsweetened)
- 1 tsp dry Coffee (Instant Powder)
- 2 oz or 1 scoops Chocolate Whey Protein
- 3 large Eggs (Whole)

Directions
1. Heat oven to 350°F. Spray mini muffin tins with cooking spray.

2. Process almonds in a food processor in pulses until finely ground. Add soy flour and baking powder; pulse to combine.
3. In a large bowl, beat butter and sugar substitute with an electric mixer until fluffy, about 2 minutes. Beat in cocoa powder, coffee powder, and 2 oz protein powder. Add eggs one at a time. Mix in almond mixture with a spatula. Divide batter in muffin tins, filling each 2/3 full. Bake 20 minutes, until set.

Nutritional Information

- Protein : 6.3g
- Fat : 9.6g
- Fiber : 1.2g
- Calories :122

Chocolate-Coconut Haystacks

Servings: 32 | Prep: 15 m | Style: American | Cook: 12 m

Ingredients

- 2 large Egg Whites
- 1 cup Sucralose Based Sweetener (Sugar Substitute)
- 2 tbsps Cocoa Powder (Unsweetened)
- 16 oz Dried Coconut
- 2 tbsps Sugar Free Chocolate Syrup

Directions

1. Heat oven to 325°F. Line baking sheets with aluminum foil.
2. Whip egg whites on low until medium peaks form; gradually beat in sugar substitute and cocoa powder; continue beating until stiff peaks form. Fold in coconut and syrup.
3. Drop mixture by rounded teaspoonfuls onto prepared baking sheets. Shape into little pyramids with wet fingertips. Bake

12 minutes. Cool on sheets 1 minute before transferring to wire racks to cool completely.

Nutritional Information

- Protein : 0.7g
- Fat : 3.3g
- Fiber : 1g
- Calories :38

Chocolate-Cream Frosty

Servings: 32 | Prep: 15 m | Style: American | Cook: 12 m

Ingredients

- 1/2 cup Tap Water
- 2 tbsps Heavy Cream
- 2 tbsps Sugar Free Chocolate Syrup

Directions

1. Place water, cream and syrup in a blender along with 3 ice cubes and blend until frothy.

Nutritional Information

- Protein : 1.6g
- Fat : 11.1g
- Fiber : 1g
- Calories :119

Chocolate-Ginger Cake

Servings: 16 | Prep: 20 m | Style: Other | Cook: 45 m

Ingredients

- 1/3 second spray Original Canola Cooking Spray
- 3/4 cup half Pecans
- 4 oz Unsweetened Baking Chocolate Squares
- 1/3 cup Tap Water
- 1/3 cup Canola Vegetable Oil
- 1/4 cup Cocoa Powder (Unsweetened)
- 1/4 cup dry Whole Grain Soy Flour
- 2 1/4 cups Sucralose Based Sweetener (Sugar Substitute)
- 12 large Eggs (Whole)
- 2 tsps Ginger (Ground)
- 1/4 tsp Cream Of Tartar

Directions

1. Preheat over to 350°F. Toast pecans in an even layer on a cookie sheet for 8 minutes. Cool, coarsely chop the pecans and set aside.
2. Lower oven to 325°F. Grease the bottom of a 10-inch tube pan, and line with parchment or waxed paper.
3. Place chocolate and the water in a microwavable bowl; microwave on high 1 to 2 minutes, until chocolate is melted, checking at 1-minute intervals. Stir until smooth, cool to lukewarm, then stir in oil; set aside.
4. In a food processor, pulse pecans, cocoa powder and soy flour until pecans are finely ground. In a large bowl, beat egg yolks with cup sugar substitute on high speed with an electric mixer, until light and fluffy, about 5 minutes. Stir in melted chocolate, pecan mixture and ginger.
5. In another large bowl, beat egg whites and cream of tartar on medium-high speed with an electric mixer, until frothy. Gradually add remaining sugar substitute, beating until stiff peaks form. With a rubber spatula, fold one-third of the meringue into the yolk mixture to lighten; fold in the remaining meringue until just combined.

6. Pour batter evenly in prepared pan and bake until a toothpick inserted in center of cake comes out clean, about 45 minutes. Allow cake to cool for 30 minutes before removing from pan.
7. To remove: Run a knife around the inner and outer rim of cake, place a wire rack or plate over pan, and invert. Remove pan, and peel off paper. Cool completely before cutting into 16 servings.

Nutritional Information
- Protein : 6.6g
- Fat : 15.6g
- Fiber : 2.2g
- Calories :185

Chocolate-Mint Mousse Layer Cake

Servings: 8 | Prep: 180 m | Style: Other | Cook: 25 m

Ingredients
- 1/3 second spray Original Canola Cooking Spray
- 1 cup Heavy Cream
- 2 tsps Vanilla Extract
- 1/2 oz Coffee (Instant Powder)
- 1 1/4 cup dries Whole Grain Soy Flour
- 1/2 cup Cocoa Powder (Unsweetened)
- 1/2 cup half Pecans
- 1/2 tsp Baking Powder (Straight Phosphate, Double Acting)
- 1/2 tsp Salt
- 1 cup Unsalted Butter Stick
- 1 cup Sucralose Based Sweetener (Sugar Substitute)
- 8 servings Chocolate Mint Mousse

- 4 large Eggs (Whole)

Directions

Use the Atkins recipe for Chocolate-Mint Mousse (See recipe).

1. Preheat oven to 325°F. Grease two 8 round cake pans with oil spray.
2. In a small bowl, mix cream, vanilla and coffee. Set aside. In a medium bowl, whisk together soy flour, cocoa, pecans, baking powder and salt. Set aside. In a large bowl, with an electric mixer on medium speed, beat butter with half of the sugar substitute until light and fluffy, about 5 minutes. Separate the eggs into yolks and whites. Add egg yolks, one at a time, beating well and scraping down the sides of the bowl after each addition. Add heavy cream mixture and beat until well-blended. Turn mixer speed down to low, and slowly add dry ingredients, one third at a time, beating until just-combined. Set aside.
3. In another large bowl, beat egg whites until soft peaks form, about 3 minutes. Add remaining sugar substitute and beat until stiff peaks, about 1 more minute. Using a rubber spatula, fold whites into chocolate batter in three parts, combining thoroughly after each addition.
4. Divide batter in prepared pans; smooth tops. Bake 20 minutes, or until cake springs back when touched in the middle. Cool in pans on racks 5 minutes; invert onto racks to cool completely, about 2 hours.
5. To assemble cake: Cut off rounded tops of each cake. Place one cake layer on a serving plate, cut side down. Spread top with half of mousse filling, leaving a 1/2 border. Place cut side of the other cake layer down on top of the mousse, pressing gently, being careful not to let mousse squirt out. Top this with remaining mousse and swirl decoratively. Garnish with raspberries and mint leaves. Makes 8 servings.

Nutritional Information

- Protein : 11.8g
- Fat : 66.8g
- Fiber : 4.4g
- Calories :703

Chocolate-Peanut Whip

Servings: 1 | Prep: 5 m | Style: American

Ingredients

- 1 tbsp Cocoa Powder (Unsweetened)
- 1 tbsp Natural Creamy Peanut Butter 1/3 Less Sodium & Sugar
- 2 tsps Sucralose Based Sweetener (Sugar Substitute)
- 2 tbsps Heavy Cream

Directions

1. Using a spatula, blend together 1 Tbsp unsweetened cocoa powder, 1 Tbsp smooth peanut butter and 1 packet of sweetener.
2. Whip 2 Tbsp heavy cream until soft peaks form.
3. Gently fold into the peanut butter mix. This is also delicious with almond butter instead of peanut butter.

Nutritional Information

- Protein : 5.7g
- Fat : 19.9g
- Fiber : 2.7g
- Calories :214

Chunky Mocha Ice Cream

Servings: 8 | Prep: 240 m | Style: American | Cook: 5 m

Ingredients

- 1 tsp Gelatin Powder (Unsweetened)
- 1 cup Tap Water
- 6 large Egg Yolks
- 1 cup Sucralose Based Sweetener (Sugar Substitute)
- 2 1/2 cups Heavy Cream
- 1/2 cup Cocoa Powder (Unsweetened)
- 4 tsp roundeds Coffee (Instant Powder, Decaffeinated)
- 1 tsp Vanilla Extract
- 1/2 tsp Salt
- 3 bars Snack Caramel Double Chocolate Crunch Bar

Directions

1. Sprinkle gelatin over water and let soften, about 5 minutes.
2. In a medium bowl, whisk yolks and sugar substitute to combine.
3. In a medium pot, mix cream, gelatin mixture, cocoa powder and coffee. Cook over medium-low heat, stirring occasionally, until cocoa and coffee granules have dissolved and mixture has begun to simmer.
4. Slowly pour 1 cup of hot cocoa mixture over egg yolk mixture, whisking constantly. Pour mixture back into pot. Cook, stirring constantly, until mixture is thick enough to coat the back of a spoon. Remove from heat. Stir in vanilla and salt. Chill mixture 4 hours.
5. Pour mixture into ice cream maker. Process according to manufacturer's directions. About 5 minutes before ice cream is finished, add the chopped bars.

Nutritional Information

- Protein : 9.1g
- Fat : 35.2g
- Fiber : 5.9g
- Calories :389

Cinnamon Custard

Servings: 6 | Prep: 20 m | Style: Mexican | Cook: 30 m

Ingredients
- 2 cups Heavy Cream
- 1/2 tsp Cinnamon
- 2 large Eggs (Whole)
- 1/2 cup Sucralose Based Sweetener (Sugar Substitute)
- 1/8 tsp Salt
- 1/2 tsp Vanilla Extract
- 6 tbsps Caramel Sugar Free Syrup
- 2 large Egg Yolks

Directions

This delectable Mexican dessert can be prepared a day ahead, covered with plastic wrap and refrigerated.

1. In a medium-size heavy saucepan, combine cream and cinnamon. Heat over medium heat, whisking constantly to thoroughly blend cinnamon into cream, just until cream begins to steam. Do not boil. Remove from heat.
2. Heat oven to 300°F.
3. In a medium bowl, whisk eggs, egg yolks, sugar substitute and salt together until pale yellow and slightly thickened.

4. Using a soup ladle and whisking constantly, very gradually pour in the hot cream. When all the cream has been added, whisk in the vanilla extract.
5. Pour about 1/2 cup of the cream mixture into each of six 4-ounce custard cups (or pour entire mixture into a 2-quart round baking dish).
6. Place the cups or baking dish in a roasting pan. Carefully pour enough boiling water(about 4 cups) in the roasting pan to come halfway up the sides of the cups or baking dish.
7. Bake until custard is still slightly loose in center, about 30 minutes. (Bake the baking dish about 5 minutes more).
8. Using an oven mitt, carefully remove cups from water bath.
9. Serve warm, at room temperature or cold, toping each serving with 1 tablespoon of caramel syrup.

Nutritional Information
- Protein : 4.5g
- Fat : 32.6g
- Fiber : 0.1g
- Calories :327

Cinnamon-Almond Meringues

Servings: 8 | Prep: 120 m | Style: French | Cook: 90 m

Ingredients
- 1/2 cup whole Almonds
- 10 individual packets Sucralose Based Sweetener (Sugar Substitute)
- 3 large Egg Whites
- 1/2 tsp Pure Almond Extract
- 1/2 tsp Cinnamon
- 1/8 tsp Cream Of Tartar

Directions

This recipe is suitable for all phases except the first two weeks of Induction due to the almonds.

1. Heat oven to 200°F. Line a baking sheet with aluminum foil.
2. In a food processor, chop nuts with sugar substitute until nuts are finely ground.
3. In a large bowl, with electric mixer at high speed, beat egg whites until soft peaks form. Add the cream of tartar, almond extract and cinnamon beating until stiff peaks form. Gently fold in nut mixture.
4. With a spoon, drop 8 evenly spaced mounds onto prepared baking sheet. Make a depression in center of each with the back of the spoon. Bake meringues on center oven rack 1½ hours, until golden and very dry. Turn off oven and let meringues dry in oven until cool. Carefully peel meringues off foil.

Nutritional Information
- Protein : 3.3g
- Fat : 4.4g
- Fiber : 1.2g
- Calories :64

Classic Apple Tart

Servings: 8 | Prep: 30 m | Style: American | Cook: 45 m

Ingredients
- 5 medium (2-3/4" dia) (approx 3 per lb) Apples (Without Skin)

- 1/4 cup Sucralose Based Sweetener (Sugar Substitute)
- 3/4 tsp Cinnamon
- 1/8 tsp Nutmeg (Ground)
- 1 serving Atkins Cuisine Pie Crust
- 1 tbsp Unsalted Butter Stick

Directions

1. Prepare Atkins Cuisine Pie Crust (see recipe) and press evenly into a 10-inch tart pan with removable bottom. Freeze 15 minutes.
2. Heat oven to 350°F. In a large bowl, combine apples, sugar substitute, cinnamon and nutmeg. Toss until apples are evenly coated. Spoon into crust; dot top with butter.
3. Bake tart 30 minutes. Cover loosely with foil and bake 10 to 20 minutes more, until apples are tender when pierced with the tip of a knife. Cool tart on wire rack.
4. Serve warm or at room temperature, with ice cream and praline sauce, if desired.

Nutritional Information

- Protein : 8.2g
- Fat : 14.3g
- Fiber : 3.1g
- Calories :238

Classic Chocolate Cupcakes

Servings: 12 | Prep: 10 m | Style: American | Cook: 22 m

Ingredients

- 1 cup Unsalted Butter Stick
- 9 tbsps Xylitol
- 3 large Eggs (Whole)
- 4 tsps Vanilla Extract

- 5 fl ozs Heavy Cream
- 3 tbsps Tap Water
- 2 tbsps Organic High Fiber Coconut Flour
- 1 cup Blanched Almond Flour
- 1/3 cup Cocoa Powder (Unsweetened)
- 1/2 tsp Baking Powder (Straight Phosphate, Double Acting)
- 1/4 tsp Baking Soda
- 1/4 tsp Salt
- 2 oz Unsweetened Baking Chocolate Squares
- 1 tsp dry Coffee (Instant Powder)

Directions

Cupcakes:

1. Preheat oven to 325°F. Line a muffin tin with 12 paper or foil liners.
2. Beat 1/2 cup softened butter with 5 tablespoons xylitol until light and fluffy; about 3 minutes. Add the eggs one at a time until fully incorporated, then add 3 tsp vanilla, 2oz (about 1/4 cup) heavy cream, water and coconut flour. Blend thoroughly.
3. In a sepatate bowl whisk to combine the almond flour, cocoa powder, baking powder, baking soda and salt. Add to the wet ingredients and beat until smooth and thick. Divide into the muffin liners and bake for 20-25 minutes or until fully cooked, be careful not to over bake or they will be bitter. Allow to cool in the muffin tin for 5 minutes then transfer to a baking rack to cool.

Frosting:

1. Melt the chocolate with 3oz (about 1/3 cup) heavy cream in the microwave at 20 second intervals. Stir and allow to cool

completely. Once cooled whisk in 4 tablespoons xylitol. Set aside.
2. In a very small bowl stir to combine the 1 tsp vanilla, 1 tsp cocoa powder (optional) and 1 tsp instant coffee. Set aside.
3. Transfer cooled chocolate to a medium bowl and beat with the remaining 1/2 cup butter on medium speed until lighter in color and fluffy. Add the reserved vanilla mixture and beat to combine.
4. Using a piping bag and fancy tip or simply a quart-sized plastic bag with a corner cut off, pipe the frosting onto the cupcakes. Garnish with an Atkins Endulge Chocolate Peanut Candy if desired.

Nutritional Information

- Protein : 8.2g
- Fat : 28.8g
- Fiber : 12g
- Calories :311

Coconut Cookies

Servings: 12 | Prep: 8 m | Style: American | Cook: 27 m

Ingredients

- 1/3 second spray Original Canola Cooking Spray
- 1/2 cup Whole Grain Soy Flour
- 1/3 cup Dried Coconut
- 1/4 cup whole Hazelnuts or Filberts
- 2 large Egg Whites
- 1/8 can Seltzer Water
- 1 1/2 tsps Coconut Extract
- 1/2 tsp Vanilla Extract
- 1/2 tsp Salt
- 8 tbsps Unsalted Butter Stick

- 7 tbsps Sucralose Based Sweetener (Sugar Substitute)

Directions

1. Preheat oven to 350°F. Toast hazelnuts in an even layer on a cookie sheet for 8 minutes. Cool, coarsely chop and set aside.
2. Increase oven temperature to 375°F. Grease baking sheet with cooking spray.
3. In large bowl, combine soy flour, unsweetened coconut, hazelnuts, egg whites, 2 Tbsp seltzer, 1 1/2 tsp coconut and 1/2 tsp vanilla extract., salt, butter and sugar substitute. Mix well.
4. Drop by rounded 1 tablespoonful (12 cookies) onto prepared baking sheet. Bake 20 minutes, or until light golden brown. Cool cookies on baking sheet 1 minute before transferring to wire racks to cool completely.

Nutritional Information

- Protein : 2.8g
- Fat : 12.4g
- Fiber : 1.3g
- Calories :134

Coconut Lemon Ice Cream With Blackberry-Peach Compote

Servings: 8 | Prep: 480 m | Style: American | Cook: 10 m

Ingredients

- 1 pinch Stevia
- 1/2 cup Xylitol
- 3 cups Coconut Cream

- 1/16 tsp Salt
- 4 large Egg Yolks
- 1/2 cup Lemon Juice
- 4 servings Blackberry-Peach Compote

Directions

1. Use the Atkins recipe to make Blackberry-Peach Compote. The recipe suggests 4 servings of the compote, 1 serving is 1/4 cup. Based on the serving size recommended for the ice cream, it is suggested to use only 2 tablespoons of the compote for each serving. If you would like to add more please add 2.1g NC for each additional 2 tablespoons of compote to the NC value listed for this recipe.
2. Combine 2 cups coconut cream and a pinch of salt in a medium sauce pan. Heat until almost boiling. While the coconut cream is heating, combine the egg yolks, granular sugar substitutes and lemon zest. Whisk to combine.
3. Slowly pour the coconut cream into the egg yolk mixture while whisking continuously. Once incorporated transfer mixture back to the sauce pan over medium-high heat. Cook while stirring continuously until it reaches 170°F and begins to coat the back of a wooden spoon, do not allow the mixture to boil.
4. Set mixture over an ice water bath and stir in the remaining 1 cup coconut cream and 1/2 cup lemon juice. Cool to room temperature then transfer to the refrigerator. Keep in the refrigerator overnight or at least 4 hours to intensify flavors and chill properly.
5. Once chilled, place into ice cream maker and follow manufacturers instructions to make ice cream. Enjoy immediately or put into a freezer-safe container and freeze for at least 4 hours or up to one month. Makes about 1 quart of ice cream, 1 serving is about 1/2 cup. Before serving place in the refrigerator 20-30 minutes. To serve, dip ice

cream scoop into hot water and dish up ice cream. Top with 2 tablespoons Blackberry-Peach Compote.

Nutritional Information

- Protein : 3.2g
- Fat : 15.9g
- Fiber : 13.8g
- Calories :214

Coconut Macaroons

Servings: 30 | Prep: 20 m | Style: American | Cook: 12 m

Ingredients

- 1/3 second spray Original Canola Cooking Spray
- 4 large Egg Whites
- 2/3 cup Sucralose Based Sweetener (Sugar Substitute)
- 1/2 tsp Vanilla Extract
- 1/4 tsp Salt
- 2 cups Dried Coconut

Directions

1. Heat oven to 325°F. Spray two baking sheets with oil spray.
2. With an electric mixer on medium speed, beat egg whites until medium peaks form. Gradually beat in sugar substitute, vanilla extract and salt. Turn speed up to high and continue beating until stiff (but not dry) peaks form.
3. Using a rubber spatula, fold in coconut.
4. Drop tablespoon-sized mounds of mixture onto prepared baking sheets. Bake 15 minutes. Cool on sheets 1 minute before carefully transferring to wire racks to cool completely.

Nutritional Information

- Protein : 0.8g

- Fat : 3.5g
- Fiber : 0.9g
- Calories :40

Coconut Panna Skullotta

Servings: 12 | Prep: 240 m | Style: American

Ingredients

- 1 14 oz can Coconut Cream
- 2 oz Gelatin Powder (Unsweetened)
- 2 cups Heavy Cream
- 1/2 cup Sucralose Based Sweetener (Sugar Substitute)
- 1 tsp Vanilla Extract
- 2 tsps Coconut Extract

Directions

1. Plastic skull molds can be found at hobby stores in the baking section and during seasonal promotions. Cake pans also work nicely, just be sure your mold will hold 4 fluid cups.
2. Pour 1 cup of the coconut milk into a medium bowl. Sprinkle with the gelatin and let stand until softened, about 1 minute
3. In a small saucepan, combine the remaining coconut milk with the cream. Heat over medium heat, stirring, until small bubbles begin to form along the sides of the pan. Pour over the gelatin mixture. Stir in sucralose and mix well. Allow to cool to room temperature.
4. Once the mixture has cooled, stir in the vanilla and 2 tsp coconut extract. Spray a 4-cup mold with cooking spray, pour in the gelatin mixture, cover with plastic wrap and refrigerate overnight or until set; at least 4 hours. To serve, pull the panna cotta away from the mold at the edges then

carefully invert onto a plate. Garnish with unsweetened shredded coconut if desired.

Nutritional Information

- Protein : 2.5g
- Fat : 21.6g
- Fiber : 0g
- Calories :212

Coconut Shortcakes With Berries And Cream

Servings: 6 | Prep: 20 m | Style: American | Cook: 12 m

Ingredients

- 1/4 cup Whole Grain Soy Flour
- 1 tsp Baking Powder (Straight Phosphate, Double Acting)
- 6 tbsp raws Unsweetened Shredded Coconut
- 4 tbsps Sucralose Based Sweetener (Sugar Substitute)
- 3 tbsps Unsalted Butter Stick
- 1 large Egg (Whole)
- 1 tsp Coconut Extract
- 1 2/3 cups Heavy Cream
- 1 tsp Vanilla Extract
- 1 1/4 cups Red Raspberries
- 1 1/4 cups Strawberries
- 1/2 cup Blueberries

Directions

1. Heat oven to 375°F. In a large mixer bowl, combine soy flour, baking powder, ¼ cup coconut, 3 tablespoons sugar substitute and the melted butter. Make a well in center and add egg, coconut extract and 2/3 cup heavy cream. Whisk the liquid ingredients together until blended, then combine with the dry mixture, mixing just until blended.
2. Drop the mixture by slightly rounded ¼ cupfuls onto a baking sheet to make 6 mounds. Using fingertips, shape each into 2½ rounds; divide and sprinkle remaining coconut over tops. Cover with plastic wrap and refrigerate 20 minutes. Bake 12 minutes, until lightly golden around edges and firm to the touch. Transfer to a wire rack and cool completely.
3. Meanwhile, with an electric mixer on medium-high, beat together remaining 1 cup heavy cream, 1 tablespoon sugar substitute and the vanilla extract to soft peaks. Whisk 1 tbsp sugar-free jam (if using) in a medium bowl until smooth; add raspberries, sliced strawberries and blueberries, tossing gently until coated.
4. To serve, split the shortcakes in half horizontally. Spread 1/3 cup whipped cream on the bottom of each shortcake. Spoon ½ cup of the berries over whipped cream and cover with shortcake top. Top with a dollop of whipped cream, if desired.

Nutritional Information
- Protein : 8.2g
- Fat : 37.2g
- Fiber : 4.7g
- Calories :422

Coconut-Cashew Chocolate Truffles

Servings: 32 | Prep: 10 m | Style: French

Ingredients

- 3/4 cup Heavy Cream
- 2 tbsps Sucralose Based Sweetener (Sugar Substitute)
- 2 tbsps Unsalted Butter Stick
- 14 oz Sugar Free Chocolate Chips
- 3 oz Unsweetened Baking Chocolate Squares
- 3/4 tsp Vanilla Extract
- 8 oz Dried Coconut
- 1/2 cup Organic Raw Cashews

Directions

1. Combine cream, sugar substitute and butter in a small saucepan. Bring to a simmer. Place chopped chocolate in a medium bowl; pour hot cream mixture over chocolate. Let stand 5 minutes.
2. Stir chocolate mixture gently until chocolate is completely melted. Stir in extract and 1/2 cup of the coconut. Refrigerate until firm, about 1 hour 45 minutes, stirring occasionally (Truffles will be easier to form if the mixture is not too stiff).
3. Toast the remaining 1/2 cup coconut in a dry skillet over medium heat, shaking often, until lightly browned; transfer to a bowl and cool.
4. Roll the chocolate mixture into 32 balls about the size of large marbles. Roll half of the balls in cashews and half in toasted coconut. Place in an airtight container between layers of wax paper. Can refrigerate up to one week.

Nutritional Information

- Protein : 1.1g
- Fat : 8.8g
- Fiber : 1.4g
- Calories :93

Coconut-Lime Mousse

Servings: 4 | **Prep:** 10 m | **Style:** American

Ingredients

- 2 oz Cream Cheese
- 4 individual packets Sucralose Based Sweetener (Sugar Substitute)
- 1/4 cup Fresh Lime Juice
- 1 tsp Vanilla Extract
- 1 cup Heavy Cream

Directions

1. Using an electric mixer, beat together 2 oz soft cream cheese and 4 packets of granular sugar substitute (equivalent to 8 teaspoons) until smooth.
2. Slowly add 1/4 cup lime juice, beating until creamy.
3. Beat in 1 teaspoon coconut extract (vanilla may be used if coconut is unavailable) and 1 cup heavy cream until fluffy.
4. Place in four bowls, sprinkle with 1 Tbsp unsweetened coconut flakes each (optional, don't forget to add in .4g NC carbs) and refrigerate until serving.

Nutritional Information

- Protein : 2.1g
- Fat : 27.1g
- Fiber : 0.1g
- Calories :266

Coeur A La Creme

Servings: 6 | Prep: 720 m | Style: French

Ingredients

- 4 oz Cream Cheese
- 1/4 cup, small curd (not packed) Cottage Cheese
- 1/4 cup Sour Cream (Cultured)
- 1/2 cup Heavy Cream
- 4 tsps Sucralose Based Sweetener (Sugar Substitute)
- 1 tsp Vanilla Extract
- 1/8 tsp Salt

Directions

1. To prepare molds: Poke several holes in bottoms of disposable muffin tins. Wet cheesecloth, wring out and fold in half. Drape cheesecloth over tin and press into molds, leaving a 2-inch overhang along border of tin. Set aside.
2. To prepare Coeur: In a food processor, pulse cream cheese, cottage cheese and sour cream until smooth, scraping sides occasionally as needed. Transfer to large bowl and set aside.
3. In another medium bowl, with an electric mixer on medium-high speed, whip cream, sugar substitute, vanilla and salt until stiff peaks form, about 4 minutes. In three additions, fold whipped cream into cheese mixture.
4. Divide among tins, cover with overhanging cheesecloth. Place tin on rack over baking sheet. Refrigerate for 12 to 24 hours or until solid. If desired, serve with a berry purée, sweetened with sugar substitute.

Nutritional Information

- Protein : 2.8g
- Fat : 15.8g
- Fiber : 0g
- Calories :161

Coffee Eggnog

Servings: 4 | Prep: 5 m | Style: Other

Ingredients
- 1 tsp Sucralose Based Sweetener (Sugar Substitute)
- 1/2 tsp Vanilla Extract
- 1 cup (8 fl oz) Coffee (Brewed From Grounds, Decaffeinated)
- 1 cup Heavy Cream
- 4 fl oz (no ice) Rum
- 2 large Eggs (Whole)
- 1/8 tsp Cinnamon

Directions
1. In a small bowl, beat eggs and sugar substitute. Add vanilla, coffee, cream and rum (if using); mix thoroughly.
2. Sprinkle top with cinnamon. Enjoy!

Nutritional Information
- Protein : 4.3g
- Fat : 24.5g
- Fiber : 0g
- Calories :308

Cranberry Parfait

Servings: 8 | Prep: 180 m | Style: French

Ingredients
- 1 cup whole Cranberries
- 8 oz Sugar Free French Vanilla Syrup
- 2 scoops Vanilla Whey Protein

- 3 cups Tap Water
- 2 1/2 package (1 oz) Gelatin Powder (Unsweetened)
- 4 individual packets Sucralose Based Sweetener (Sugar Substitute)

Directions

1. In a blender, combine cranberries, vanilla syrup and shake mix. Purée until smooth.
2. In a mixing bowl, pour 1 cup cold water; sprinkle gelatin into water and let stand 1 minute.
3. Combine remaining 2 cups water with sugar substitute and bring to a boil (either in a microwave or on the stovetop). Add hot water mixture to gelatin mixture; stir until gelatin dissolves.
4. Add berry mixture and stir until smooth. Pour into eight custard cups. Chill at least 3 hours to set.

Nutritional Information

- Protein : 7.4g
- Fat : 0g
- Fiber : 0.6g
- Calories :38

Cranberry-Raspberry Gelatin Dessert

Servings: 6 | Prep: 180 m | Style: American

Ingredients

- 2 package (1 oz) Gelatin Powder (Unsweetened)
- 1/2 cup Tap Water
- 2 cup (8 fl oz) Low Calorie Cranberry Juice Drink with Vitamin C Added
- 8 tbsps Raspberry Sugar Free Syrup
- 2 tsps Fresh Lemon Juice

Directions

1. Place gelatin in a large bowl. Bring water to a boil. Pour water over gelatin; stir until dissolved.
2. Add cranberry juice, raspberry syrup, and lemon juice. Mix well.
3. Divide mixture in 6 dessert glasses. Chill until gelled, about 3 hours.

Nutritional Information

- Protein : 2g
- Fat : 0g
- Fiber : 0g
- Calories :23

Part 2

Introduction

I want to thank you and congratulate you for buying this book, this book- how do you start on this book. This is the question that most people have. The greatest challenge is not usually the zeal and the motivation to start on this books but rather how to get easy and delicious recipes to get started on those books.

We have been made to believe that you have not eaten any meal unless you have some grains. However do you know that some of these grains are the reason for all the problems that we are currently facing like besity. This books has amazing recipes to get you started on your journey to eating like caveman;

I have compiled breakfast, lunch, dinner and dessert recipes with this books be rest assured that you will have no problem starting this book recipes. As the books recipes are simple, easy to make and delicious. Thanks again for downloading this books, I hope you enjoy it.

Apricot-Glazed Roasted Asparagus (Low Fat)

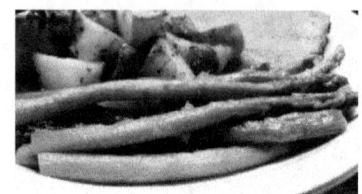

Ingredients

- 1 lb fresh asparagus spear (ends trimmed)
- 3 tablespoons apricot preserves
- 1 tablespoon soy sauce
- 1/8-1/4 teaspoon garlic powder
- 1/4 teaspoon salt
- black pepper

Directions

Rinse spears under cold water then pat dry with paper towels.

Set oven to 375 degrees.

Grease a large baking sheet.

In a small bowl combine the apricot preserves with soy sauce, garlic powder and salt; pour over the asparagus on the baking sheet and toss using hands to coat with the mixture.

Bake for about 10-15 minutes or until the asparagus is crisp-tender.

Season with freshly ground black pepper to taste.

Quick Low-Fat Mushrooms

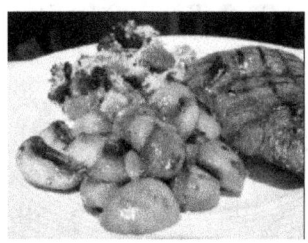

Ingredients
- 1 tablespoon olive oil
- 1 garlic clove, crushed
- 1 medium sized onion, finely diced
- 1 tablespoon chicken stock powder or 2 crumbled chicken stock cubes
- 1/2 teaspoon dried basil
- 500 g button mushrooms, halved .or quartered with stems removed
- 1 tablespoon olive oil, extra only if required
- salt
- pepper
- 1/4 cup water
- 2 teaspoons cornflour (US cornstarch)

Directions

Heat the oil in a non-stick frying pan over medium heat.

Add the garlic and onion -stir until the onion has softened. Add the stock powder and dried basil. This should take roughly 3 minutes.

Add the cut mushrooms and continue to cook for another minute. Add the extra oil if required to moisten the mushrooms. Season with salt and pepper to taste.

Mix the cornflour with a little water in your measuring cup. Add more water to bring to the 1/4 cup measurement of water. Mix and add over the mushrooms. You can use cream or evaporated milk in place of the water if you wish.

Continue to cook and stir until done to your liking. I prefer to keep my mushrooms chunky.

Serve over toast, steak or chicken.

Very Simple Oven Fried Chicken -- Low Fat

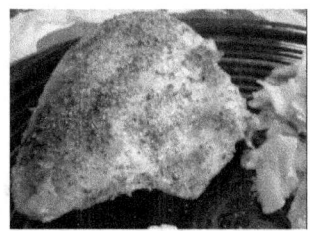

Ingredients

- 2 skinless chicken breast halves, bone in
- vegetable oil cooking spray
- 1/2 teaspoon salt
- 1/4 teaspoon pepper, freshly ground
- 1 teaspoon paprika

Directions

Preheat oven to 400 degrees Fahrenheit.

Sprinkle salt and pepper over both sides of chicken.

Spray chicken all over with veggies spray.

Sprinkle all over with paprika.

Fit a rack into a roasting pan; spray with veggie spray.

Place chicken bone side down on roaster rack.

Roast for approximately 45 minutes or until juices run clear.

Crustless Spinach Quiche (Low Fat)

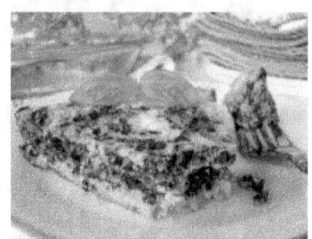

Ingredients

- 2 teaspoons canola oil
- 1 medium onion, finely chopped
- 1 (10 ounce) package frozen spinach, thawed and drained
- 1 1/2 cups light cheddar cheese (6 oz.)
- 6 large egg whites
- 1 large egg
- 1/3 cup fat-free cottage cheese
- 1/4 teaspoon cayenne pepper
- 1/8 teaspoon salt
- 1/8 teaspoon nutmeg

Directions

In a nonstick skillet over medium-high heat, heat oil.

Add onion and cook, stirring, for 5 minutes, or until translucent.

Add spinach and stir until moisture has evaporated, about 3 minutes longer.

Sprinkle cheese evenly in 9-inch pie plate coated with cooking spray.

Top with spinach mixture.

In medium bowl, whisk together egg whites, egg, cottage cheese, cayenne, salt and nutmeg.

Pour egg mixture evenly over spinach.

Bake at 375°F for 30 to 40 minutes or until set.

Let stand 5 minutes, then cut into wedges and serve.

Low Fat Spinach And Artichoke Dip

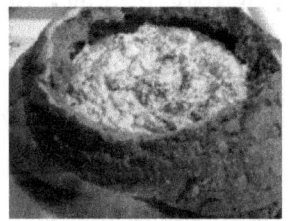

Ingredients
- 8 ounces neufchatel cheese, softened (do not use fat free)
- 1/2 cup light sour cream (do not use fat free)
- 14 ounces artichoke hearts, undrained
- 7 1/4 ounces roasted red peppers, drained
- 1/4 cup parmesan cheese, freshly grated
- 10 ounces frozen spinach,

Directions

Preheat oven to 375F and lightly spritz a shallow baking dish (1.5-2qt) with cooking spray (Pam).

Using food processor, mix light cream cheese, sour cream and artichoke hearts by pulsing until even consistency.

Add roasted bell pepper and Parmesan cheese and pulse until creamy.

To bake dip: Place mixture into prepared baking dish; add spinach and stir until combined.

Bake for 25 minutes, stirring half way through.

Dip is done when browned and bubbly around the edges.

To keep warm, lower temperature in oven to 250F and stir every 10 minutes until dip is served.

For microwave directions: Place mixture into microwave safe dish (1.5-2qt), add spinach and stir until combined.

Cover with plastic wrap, leaving room for steam to escape.
1. Microwave on HIGH for 7 minutes or until dip is hot and boiling on the sides - microwaves vary, check often.
2. Mix well before serving.

Broccoli Cheese Soup - 20 Minute Fast And Low Fat

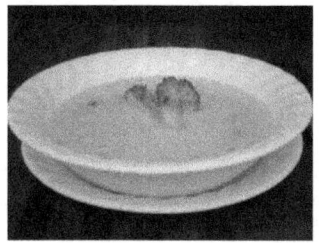

Ingredients

- 1 (1 lb) bagof frozen broccoli floret
- 1 (14 ounce) can chicken broth or 1 (14 ounce) can vegetable broth
- 2 tablespoons all-purpose flour
- 2 -4 finely chopped shallots
- 1 tablespoon butter (or 10 servings spray butter)
- 1 cup of your favorite shredded cheddar cheese (we use Kraft Cheddar Classic Melts)
- 1 cup fat-free half-and-half

Directions

Place broccoli and 3/4 cup water in microwave safe dish,

- Microwave broccoli until fork tender (about 6 min on high).

Meanwhile in sauce pan, saute shallots until clear.

When clear, add flour to pan and stir until flour cooked Add broth and 1/2 cup of broccoli water and 1/4 of broccoli spears.

Mash entire mixture with a potato masher.

Bring to a rapid boil.

Boil for about 3-5 minutes.

Decrease heat, add rest of broccoli spears (whole), half and half and cheese.

Stir until cheese melts.

Season to taste with salt and pepper and enjoy.

Lower Calorie Chicken Piccata

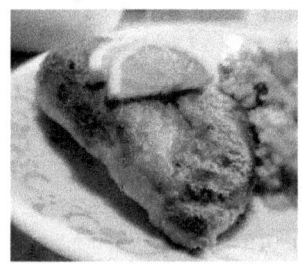

Ingredients
- 2 tablespoons Dijon mustard
- 1 large egg
- 1/2 cup dried Italian seasoned breadcrumbs
- 1 lb chicken breast
- 2 teaspoons olive oil
- 2 tablespoons chicken broth
- 1 tablespoon lemon juice
- 1 tablespoon minced parsley

- lemon, sliced (optional)

Directions

Combine the mustard and egg in a small bowl. Place the bread crumbs on a sheet of wax paper. Dip the chicken in the egg, then in the bread crumbs to cover.

Heat the oil in a large skillet over medium heat. Cook the chicken in the oil until golden and cooked through, about 5 minutes on each side. Transfer to a plate.

Add the broth and lemon juice to the skillet. Simmer 30 seconds, stir in the parsley.

Pour the sauce over the chicken and garnish with the lemon sliced, if desired.

Low Cal Dill Sauce For Poached Fish

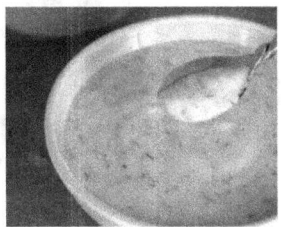

Ingredients
- 1/2 cup skim milk
- 1 teaspoon Dijon mustard

- 1/2 teaspoon salt
- 1 teaspoon minced fresh dill weed
- 1 teaspoon cornstarch
- 1 tablespoon skim milk
- 1/4-1/2 teaspoon fresh lemon juice

Directions

Mix 1/2 cup milk, mustard, salt and dill weed in a sauce pan, stir and warm over medium heat.

Mix the cornstarch with a tbsp of milk to dissolve it.

Add cornstarch to the milk, stir and bring to a slow boil, lower heat and continue to cook for 2 minutes.

Just before serving stir in lemon juice.

Low Carb Kfc Coleslaw

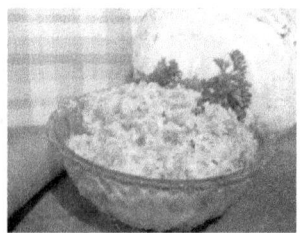

Ingredients
- 4 cups finely chopped cabbage
- 1/2 cup shredded carrot
- 4 (1 g) packages Splenda sugar substitute
- 1/2 teaspoon salt

- 1/8 teaspoon pepper
- 1/4 cup milk
- 1/2 cup mayonnaise
- 1/4 cup buttermilk
- 1 1/2 tablespoons white vinegar
- 2 1/2 tablespoons lemon juice
- 3 tablespoons minced onions

Directions

Chop the cabbage into very fine pieces about the size of rice kernels; I use the shredder on my food processor and then use the grater attachment. I find this works just perfectly.

Then I process the carrot and onion at the same time.

Dump all this into a large bowl.

Combine the Splenda, salt, pepper, milk, mayonnaise, buttermilk, vinegar, and lemon juice and whisk together until smooth.

Add the dressing to the cabbage mixture and mix well.

Cover and refrigerate for at least two hours before serving.

Chocolate Pudding, Low Fat

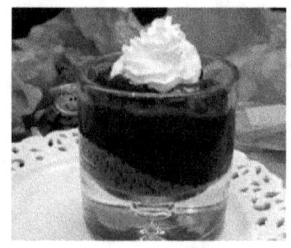

Ingredients

- cup sugar
- 1/4 cup cocoa powder
- 2 tablespoons cornstarch
- 2 cups nonfat milk
- 2 ounces bittersweet chocolate, roughly chopped
- 1 teaspoon vanilla

Directions

In a saucepan, stir together sugar, cocoa, and cornstarch; while stirring, gradually add milk and cook until thickened and bubbly, about 5 minutes.

Reduce heat to medium low and add bitterseet chocolate; cook, stirring, another 3 minutes; remove from heat and cool 5 minutes; add vanilla; pour into dessert dishes and serve or lay plastic on pudding surface and refrigerate.

Low Fat Chili Made With Fat-Free Ground Turkey, 210 Calories Per

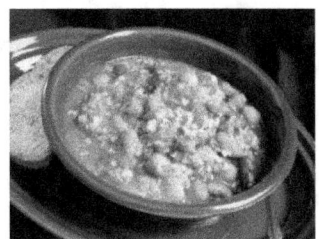

Ingredients

- cooking spray
- 3 (1 1/4 lb) packagesfat-free ground turkey
- 2 (28 ounce) cans crushed tomatoes
- 3 medium onions, diced
- 2 (1 1/4 ounce) packets taco seasoning mix, 2 packets per pound of turkey
- 3 (15 ounce) cans red kidney beans

Directions

Spray each of 3 skillets with cooking spray.

Sautee the turkey throroughly. (More effort is required stirring/separating ground-turkey "crumbles" than with high-fat, slippery ground beef.).

Lower heat. Pour off all drippings.

Add the crushed tomatoes, onions, and Taco Seasoning. Stir. Add kidney beans, stir again, and let simmer for 5 minutes.

Top with with diced tomatoes, shredded lettuce, sliced black olives & fat-free cheese if desired. Add 30 calories for each cheese slice.

Low-Fat Burgundy Beef & Vegetable Stew

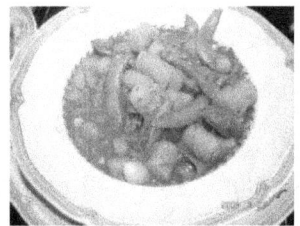

Ingredients

- 1 1/2 lbs beef eye round
- 1 tablespoon vegetable oil
- 1 teaspoon dried thyme leaves
- 1/2 teaspoon salt
- 1/2 teaspoon pepper
- 1 (13 3/4 ounce) can ready-to-serve beef broth
- 1/2 cup Burgundy wine
- 3 cloves large garlic, crushed
- 5 1/2 cups baby carrots
- 1 cup frozen whole pearl onion
- 2 tablespoons cornstarch, dissolved in 2 tablespoons water
- 1 (8 ounce) package frozen sugar snap peas

Directions

Trim fat from beef, cut into 1-inch pieces.

In Dutch oven, heat oil over medium high hunt until hot. Add beef (half at a time) and brown evenly, stirring occasionally.

Pour off drippings.

Season with thyme, salt and pepper.

Stir in broth, wine and garlic. Bring to boil; reduce heat to low.

Cover tightly and simmer 1 1/2 hours.

Add carrots and onions.

Cover and continue cooking 35 to 40 minutes or until beef and vegetables are tender.

Bring beef stew to a boil over medium-high heat. Add cornstarch mixture; cook and stir 1 minute. Stir in sugar snap peas.

1. Reduce heat to medium and cook 3 to 4 minutes or until peas are heated through.

Cauliflower Salad Made Like Potato Salad (Low Carb)

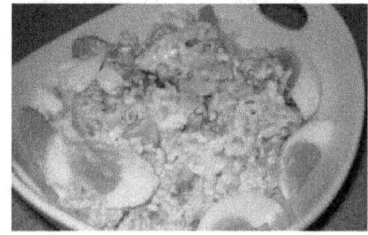

Ingredients
- 1 whole cauliflower, steamed and florets chopped into chunks

- 6 slices turkey bacon or 6 slices smoked bacon, cooked crisp and crumbled
- 4 -5 scallions, chopped
- 1/2 cup finely diced celery
- 4 hardboiled egg, peeled and chopped
- 1/3 cup regular mayonnaise
- 1/3 cup low-fat sour cream
- 1 tablespoon creole mustard
- 1/2 teaspoon kosher salt
- 1/4 teaspoon black pepper
- 1/4 teaspoon paprika

Directions

Combine ingredients and chill before serving.

Hash Browns (Patties - Low Sodium) Homemade

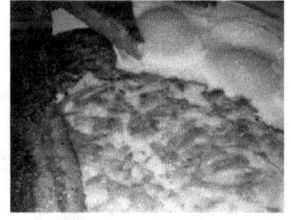

Ingredients

- 1 1/2 cups peeled and shredded potatoes
- 1/2 cup onions, minced (optional) or 1/2 cup shredded onion (optional)
- 1/2 cup egg substitute or egg, lightly beaten
- 1 1/2 tablespoons water

- 2 teaspoons Mrs. Dash seasoning mix (or other seasoning to taste)

Directions

Combine potatoes, egg substitute or eggs, water and All-Purpose Original Blend Mrs. Dash in medium bowl; mix well.

In non-stick skillet or on griddle place approximately ¼ cup potato mixture; press with spatula to about 4 inches in diameter.

Cook over medium or medium-high heat 4 to 5 minutes on each side or until golden brown.

Repeat with remaining potato mixture

Chilled Strawberry Romance: The Soup (Low Fat)

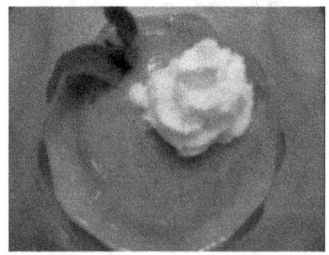

Ingredients
- 1 quart strawberry, stem tops removed
- 8 ounces non-fat vanilla yogurt
- 1 pinch ground ginger

- 1 orange, juice of
- 4-6 mint leaves

Directions

Wash and stem berries.

Place ingredients in food processor or blender and puree until smooth.

Chill and serve with a small dollop of yogurt and a mint sprig as garnish.

*It can be further enhanced with a shot of Grand Marnier or a couple ounces of sweet champagne.

Low-Fat, Low-Calorie, Jalapeno Cornbread

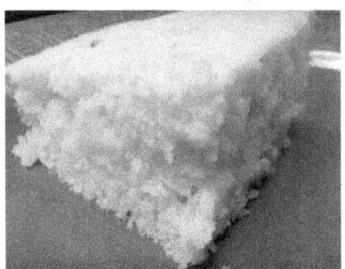

Ingredients
- 1 cup cornmeal
- 1 cup flour
- 2 tablespoons Sugar Twin (or other artificial sweetener)
- 1/4 teaspoon salt

- 1 cup soured skim milk (To make soured milk-put 1 TBSP lemon juice or vinegar in a measuring cup, then fill rest of the way)
- 1 teaspoon baking powder
- 1/2 cup crushed pineapple (drained)
- 1 egg, lightly beaten (or 2 egg whites)
- 1/4 cup jalapeno, drained and chopped

Directions

Preheat oven to 400°F; grease an 8-inch square pan or glass dish.

Combine corn meal and soured milk in a small bowl and let sit for 5 minutes. Meanwhile, combine other dry ingredients in a larger bowl.

Add crushed pineapple and egg (or egg whites) to corn meal mixture. Mix until combined.

Add corn meal mixture to dry ingredients, mix until well combined.

Add jalapenos and fold into mixture. (If it seems to thick, add a quick splash more milk and mix again).

Pour into greased pan and cook for 20-25 minutes or until a toothpick inserted in middle comes out clean and the bread is golden brown.

After cooked, slice into 9 slices and enjoy

Easiest Low Fat French Fries

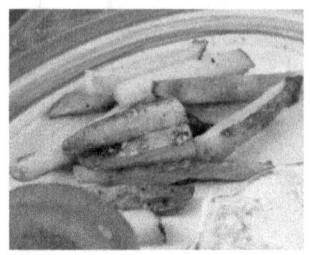

Ingredients

- 4 -6 potatoes, cut into wedges
- cooking spray
- salt and pepper

Directions

Preheat oven to 350'F.

Wash and cut potatoes into wedges.

Spray baking sheet with cooking spay.

Arrange potatoes on sheet and spray top of potatoes with cooking spray and put alittle salt and pepper on top.

Bake for 30 minutes. There is in need to turn.

enjoy.

Crustless Tomato And Basil Quiche (Low Carb)

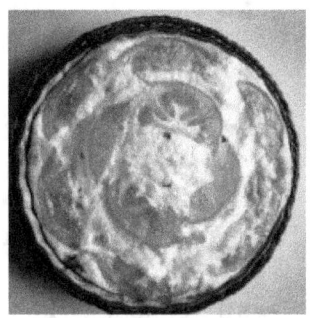

Ingredients

- 1 tablespoon olive oil
- 1 onion, sliced
- 2 cups tomatoes, sliced
- 2 tablespoons flour
- 2 teaspoons dried basil or 2 tablespoons fresh basil
- 3/4 cup egg substitute or 3 whole eggs
- 1/2 cup skim milk
- 1/2 teaspoon black pepper (or less)
- 1 cup lowfat swiss cheese, shredded

Directions

Preheat oven to 400°F.

Spray 9" pie pan with cooking spray and layer 1/2 cup of cheese on the bottom.

Heat olive oil in a large skillet over medium heat and saute onion until soft; layer over cheese in pie pan.

Sprinkle tomato slices with flour and basil, then saute 1 minute on each side; layer over onions in pie pan.

In a small bowl, whisk together eggs and milk, season with pepper and pour over the onion/tomato layers in the pie pan.

Sprinkle top of quiche with remaining 1/2 cup of cheese and bake at 400° F for 10 minutes.

Reduce heat to 350° F and bake for 15 to 20 minutes, or until filling is puffed and golden brown. Serve warm.

Fish Veronique (Low Fat, Diabetic Friendly)

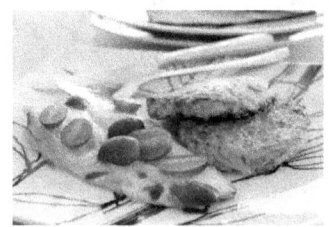

Ingredients
- 1 lb white fish fillet (cod, sole, turbot, etc.)
- 1/4 teaspoon salt
- 1/8 teaspoon black pepper

- 1/4 cup dry white wine
- 1/4 cup chicken stock or 1/4 cup broth, skim fat from top
- 1 tablespoon lemon juice
- 1 tablespoon soft margarine
- 2 tablespoons flour
- 3/4 cup skim milk or 3/4 cup 1% low-fat milk
- 1/2 cup seedless grapes

Directions

Spray 10x6-inch baking dish with nonstick spray. Place fish in pan and sprinkle with salt and pepper.

Mix wine, stock, and lemon juice in small bowl and pour over fish.

Cover and bake at 350º F for 15 minutes.

Melt margarine in small saucepan. Remove from heat and blend in flour. Gradually add milk and cook over moderately low heat, stirring constantly until thickened.

Remove fish from oven and pour liquid from baking dish into cream sauce, stirring until blended. Pour sauce over fish and sprinkle with grapes.

Broil about 4 inches from heat 5 minutes or until sauce starts to brown.

Low Carb Pizza - Zucchini "Crust"

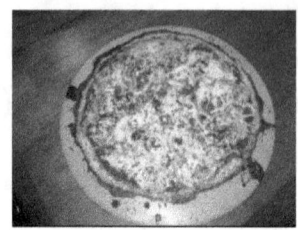

Ingredients

- 4 medium zucchini, grated
- 2 eggs
- 1 (14 ounce) jar pizza sauce
- pepperoni (or whatever your favorite pizza toppings are)
- 1 cup grated mozzarella cheese
- 1 cup grated cheddar cheese

Directions

Preheat oven to 375 degrees.

Spray a pizza pan with cooking spray.

Mix well grated zucchini and 2 eggs.

Place zucchini mixture on the pizza pan, spreading out to the edges of the pan.

Bake at 375 degrees for 30 minutes.

Spread pizza sauce on partially-cooked "crust" to within about 1/2 inch of the edge.

Top with pepperoni and/or other pizza toppings.

Sprinkle both cheeses on top.

Bake for another 30 minutes or until cheese begins to brown.

Low-Fat Scalloped Potatoes

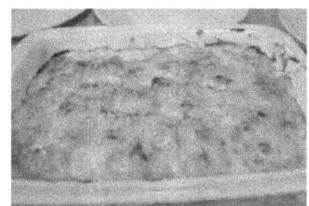

Ingredients
- 2 tablespoons unsalted butter (plus more to coat the dish)
- kosher salt
- 3 lbs yukon gold potatoes, peeled and thinly sliced
- 2 tablespoons all-purpose flour
- 1 cup low-fat milk, at room temperature (1%)
- 1 cup whole milk, at room temperature
- fresh ground pepper
- 1/4 teaspoon freshly grated nutmeg
- 1/4 cup gruyere cheese, grated

Directions

Preheat the oven to 350 degrees. Lightly butter a 3-qt baking dish. Bring a large pot of salted water to a boil; add the potatoes and cook until just tender, 8-10 minutes. Drain the potatoes and return to the pot. Meanwhile, melt 2 tablespoons butter in a saucepan over medium heat. Stir in the flour with a wooden spoon to make a paste. Cook, stirring, until the paste puffs slightly, about 1 minute. Gradually whisk in both milks and simmer, whisking constantly, until thickened, about 3 minutes. Remove from the heat and whisk in 1/2 teaspoons pepper, 1 1/2 teaspoons salt and the nutmeg. Pour the sauce over the potatoes and gently toss to coat.

Transfer the potato mixture to the prepared baking dish and sprinkle with the gruyere cheese. Bake until heated through, about 10 minutes. Switch the oven to broil the potatoes until browned on top, about 5 minutes. Let rest 10 minutes before serving.

Chewy Lower Fat Brownies

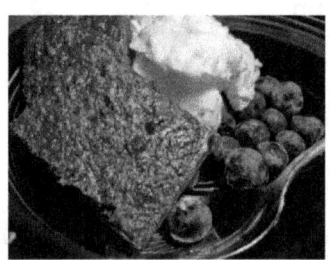

Ingredients
- 3/4 cup flour

- 1/2 cup less 1 tablespoon sugar
- 1/3 cup unsweetened cocoa
- 1/2 teaspoon baking powder
- 1/4 teaspoon salt (to taste)
- 3 tablespoons unsalted butter or 3 tablespoons reduced-calorie margarine, melted
- 1 teaspoon unsalted butter or 1 teaspoon reduced-calorie margarine, melted
- 3 large egg whites
- 1 teaspoon vanilla extract
- 1 1/2 ounces chopped walnuts

Directions

Spray an 8 inch square baking pan with non-stick cooking spray; set aside.

In large bowl, with fork, stir together flour, sugar, cocoa, and baking powder and salt.

Stir in butter, egg whites, and vanilla; mix well. Stir in walnuts.

Spoon batter into prepared pan, spreading evenly. Bake at 350 degrees for 30 to 35 minutes. Let cool. Makes 8 servings.

Low Country Zucchini And Yellow Squash

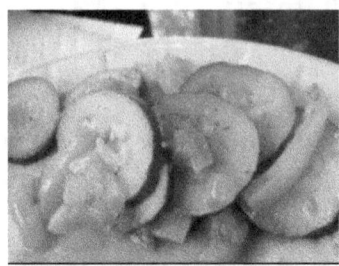

Ingredients

- 2 medium zucchini, sliced 1/4 inch thick
- 2 medium yellow squash, sliced 1/4 inch thick
- 1 sweet bell pepper, cut in 1 inch pieces
- 1 medium onion, diced
- 4 fresh tomatoes, medium size crushed (or 2 cans stewed tomatoes)
- 1/4 teaspoon dried rosemary
- 1 teaspoon salt (or to taste)
- 1/4 teaspoon black pepper
- 1 tablespoon bacon drippings (or 2 chicken bouillon cubes)

Directions

Place all ingredients in a medium saucepan and cook on medium heat, covered, 8-10 minutes.

Easy Low-Fat Creamy Dill Salmon

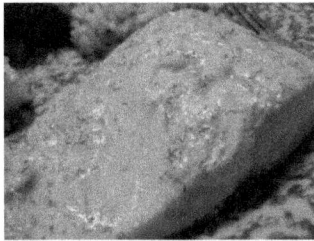

Ingredients

- 1 salmon fillet
- fat-free mayonnaise or low-fat mayonnaise or Miracle Whip
- dill
- lemon juice
- salt and pepper

Directions

Lay salmon filet on large piece of tin foil (shiny side of foil facing up).

Sprinkle salmon with lemon juice.

Spread enough mayo over salmon to cover the filet.

Season with salt and pepper.

Season with enough dill to cover the filet.

Make a "tent" around the salmon with the foil.

BBQ on medium heat until salmon is cooked to your liking.

Low-Fat Gravy

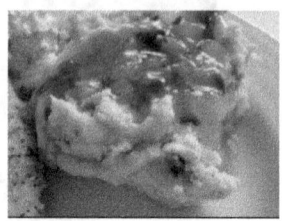

Ingredients

- 1/2 cup onion, finely chopped
- 1/2 cup mushroom, finely chopped
- 2 tablespoons fresh parsley, finely chopped
- 2 cups chicken broth, divided (reduced sodium, fat free recommended)
- 2 tablespoons cornstarch
- 1 pinch pepper

Directions

In a saucepan over medium heat, saute onion, mushroom and parsley in 1/4 cup of broth until tender.

Combine cornstarch, pepper and 1/2 cup broth, stir until smooth.

Add to saucepan along with remaining broth.

Bring to a boil, stirring occasionally.

Boil for 2 minutes.

Low-Fat Chicken With Caramelized Onions

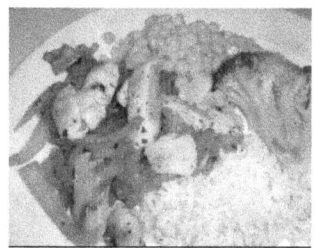

Ingredients

- /2 teaspoon salt
- 1/4 teaspoon thyme
- 1/4 teaspoon red pepper, ground
- 1/4 teaspoon black pepper
- 1 cup chicken broth
- 1/4 cup balsamic vinegar
- 1 large onion, sliced
- 1 lb boneless skinless chicken breast

Directions

Coat large skillet with cooking spray and place over medium heat until hot. Add onion.

Cover and cook 10 minutes until deep golden stirring often.

combine salt, thyme, red pepper and black pepper.

Sprinkle half the mixture over onions.

Add 1/4 cup chicken broth and cook 10 minutes, stirring frequently.

Add 6 tablespoon broth and cook until liquid evaporates.

Repeat procedure with remaining broth.

Add vinegar and cook an additional 2 minutes or until most of the liquid evaporates.

Remove from pan and keep warm.

1. Rub chicken with remaining spice mixture. Coat skillet with cooking spray and heat. Add chicken and cook for 2 minutes on each side. Serve with onions.

Chewy Lower Fat Brownies

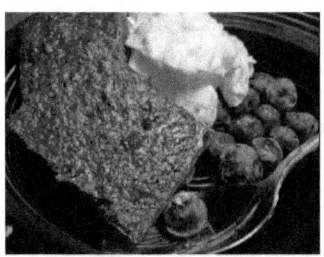

Ingredients

- 3/4 cup flour
- 1/2 cup less 1 tablespoon sugar
- 1/3 cup unsweetened cocoa
- 1/2 teaspoon baking powder
- 1/4 teaspoon salt (to taste)
- 3 tablespoons unsalted butter or 3 tablespoons reduced-calorie margarine, melted
- 1 teaspoon unsalted butter or 1 teaspoon reduced-calorie margarine, melted
- 3 large egg whites
- 1 teaspoon vanilla extract
- 1 1/2 ounces chopped walnuts

Directions

Spray an 8 inch square baking pan with non-stick cooking spray; set aside.

In large bowl, with fork, stir together flour, sugar, cocoa, and baking powder and salt.

Stir in butter, egg whites, and vanilla; mix well. Stir in walnuts.

Spoon batter into prepared pan, spreading evenly. Bake at 350 degrees for 30 to 35 minutes. Let cool. Makes 8 servings.

Low Country Zucchini And Yellow Squash

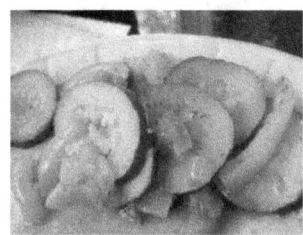

Ingredients
- 2 medium zucchini, sliced 1/4 inch thick
- 2 medium yellow squash, sliced 1/4 inch thick
- 1 sweet bell pepper, cut in 1 inch pieces
- 1 medium onion, diced
- 4 fresh tomatoes, medium size crushed (or 2 cans stewed tomatoes)
- 1/4 teaspoon dried rosemary
- 1 teaspoon salt (or to taste)
- 1/4 teaspoon black pepper
- 1 tablespoon bacon drippings (or 2 chicken bouillon cubes)

Directions

Place all ingredients in a medium saucepan and cook on medium heat, covered, 8-10 minutes.

Easy Low-Fat Creamy Dill Salmon

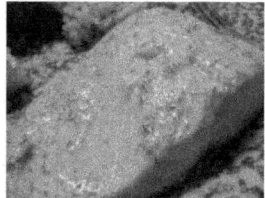

Ingredients
- 1 salmon fillet
- fat-free mayonnaise or low-fat mayonnaise or Miracle Whip
- dill
- lemon juice
- salt and pepper

Directions

Lay salmon filet on large piece of tin foil (shiny side of foil facing up).

Sprinkle salmon with lemon juice.

Spread enough mayo over salmon to cover the filet.

Season with salt and pepper.

Season with enough dill to cover the filet.

Make a "tent" around the salmon with the foil.

BBQ on medium heat until salmon is cooked to your liking.

Low-Fat Gravy

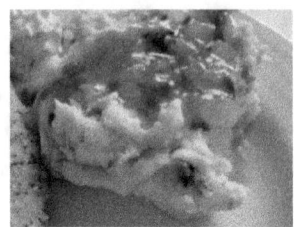

Ingredients

- 1/2 cup onion, finely chopped
- 1/2 cup mushroom, finely chopped
- 2 tablespoons fresh parsley, finely chopped
- 2 cups chicken broth, divided (reduced sodium, fat free recommended)
- 2 tablespoons cornstarch
- 1 pinch pepper

Directions

In a saucepan over medium heat, saute onion, mushroom and parsley in 1/4 cup of broth until tender.

Combine cornstarch, pepper and 1/2 cup broth, stir until smooth.

Add to saucepan along with remaining broth.

Bring to a boil, stirring occasionally.

Boil for 2 minutes.

Low-Fat Chicken With Caramelized Onions

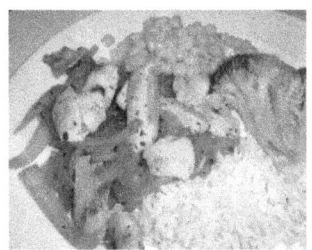

Ingredients

- 1/2 teaspoon salt
- 1/4 teaspoon thyme
- 1/4 teaspoon red pepper, ground
- 1/4 teaspoon black pepper
- 1 cup chicken broth
- 1/4 cup balsamic vinegar
- 1 large onion, sliced
- 1 lb boneless skinless chicken breast

Directions

Coat large skillet with cooking spray and place over medium heat until hot. Add onion.

Cover and cook 10 minutes until deep golden stirring often.

combine salt, thyme, red pepper and black pepper.

Sprinkle half the mixture over onions.

Add 1/4 cup chicken broth and cook 10 minutes, stirring frequently.

Add 6 tablespoon broth and cook until liquid evaporates.

Repeat procedure with remaining broth.

Add vinegar and cook an additional 2 minutes or until most of the liquid evaporates.

Remove from pan and keep warm.
1. Rub chicken with remaining spice mixture. Coat skillet with cooking spray and heat. Add chicken and cook for 2 minutes on each side. Serve with onions.

Low-Fat Carnitas

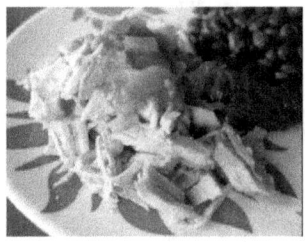

Ingredients
- 4 lbs pork loin, cut in very large pieces
- 1 1/2 quarts chicken broth
- 1 large onion, quartered
- 1 tablespoon cumin
- 1 tablespoon coriander
- 2 teaspoons oregano, dried

- 4 chipotle chiles, canned or dry
- 2 bay leaves
- to taste water
- to taste salt

Directions

To a 7- to 8-quart pan, add pork, broth, onion, coriander, cumin, oregano, chilies in sauce, sauce, and bay leaves. Add water to cover the pork.

Cover the pan and bring to a boil on high heat, then reduce heat and simmer until meat pulls apart easily with a fork, 2 to 3 hours.

Strain broth.

Cover pork with enough broth to keep moist and use remaining broth for Spiced Black Beans.

To bake carnitas, pull pork large shreds and place in a shallow baking dish.

Spoon some broth over to keep moist. Broil pork until slightly crisp (watching carefully), turn, moisten if necessary and broil again.

Low-Carb Crab Cakes

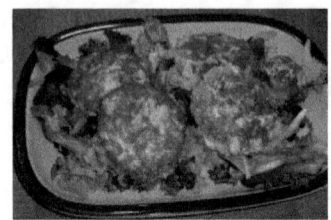

Ingredients

- 2 (6 ounce) cansfancy white crab meat, drained
- 1 egg
- 1/4 cup Italian style breadcrumbs
- 1 tablespoon parsley flakes, crushed
- 2 tablespoons mayonnaise
- 1 teaspoon Old Bay Seasoning
- 2 teaspoons Worcestershire sauce
- 1 teaspoon baking powder
- low-carb ketchup, and
- mayonnaise, for sauce

Directions

Pick over the crab meat for pieces of shell, etc.

Mix all ingredients together in a medium bowl.

(Except for Ketchup and mayonnaise for sauce.) Form into 4 patties.

Pan fry in oil over medium to medium-high heat in large non-stick skillet, Cook approximately 3 minutes on the first side before flipping for the first time.

Cook 3 minutes more on other side.

Continue cooking until both sides are golden brown.

Serve with lowcarb ketchup and mayonnaise that has some old bay seasoning mixed into it.

Low Carb Lasagna

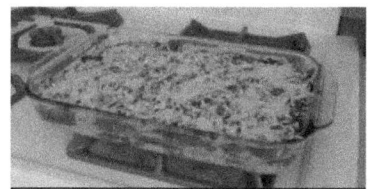

Ingredients
- 3 large zucchini
- 1 tablespoon salt
- cooking spray
- 1 1/2 cups diced onions
- 2 minced garlic cloves
- 12 ounces button mushrooms
- 3 cups chopped tomatoes
- 1 tablespoon dried basil
- 1 teaspoon dried oregano

- 1/4 teaspoon ground nutmeg
- 1/4 teaspoon black pepper
- 1/2 cup fat free mozzarella cheese
- 3 -4 cups raw spinach leaves

Directions

Slice the zucchini lengthwise into 1/8-inch thick strips. Place in a bowl and salt generously, tossing once or twice to coat well. Lay strips on paper towels on your work surface. Set aside 1 hour.

Meanwhile, spray a large saucepan with nonstick spray and set over medium heat. Add the onion; cook, stirring often, until softened, about 2 minutes. Add garlic; cook 20 seconds.

Add the mushrooms; cook, stirring often, until they give off their liquid and it reduces to a glaze, about 7 minutes.

Stir in the tomatoes, basil, oregano, nutmeg and pepper. Cook, stirring occasionally, until the tomatoes start to break down and the sauce thickens, about 25 minutes.

Position the rack in the center of the oven and preheat the oven to 350°F.

Blot any moisture off the zucchini strips with paper towels. Use one third of the zucchini strips to line the bottom of a 9 x 13-inch baking pan, laying them lengthwise like you would lasagna noodles. Top evenly with one third of the sauce, then one third of the shredded cheese. Place half the remaining zucchini strips on top, as before, then top evenly with half the remaining sauce and half the remaining cheese. Repeat this process one more time: using the remaining zucchini, remaining sauce, and remaining cheese.

Bake, uncovered, until bubbling, about 45 minutes. Let stand at room temperature for 10 minutes before slicing into 6 pieces; serve.

Low Cal Sole

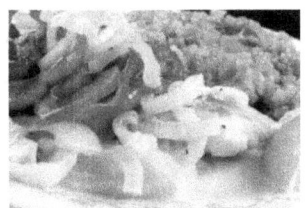

Ingredients
- 4 sole fillets
- 1 onion
- 1 green pepper
- 1 red bell pepper
- 1 garlic clove
- 1 tomatoes
- 4 tablespoons lemon juice
- salt

- lemon-pepper seasoning
- 1 tablespoon olive oil

Directions

Place the fish fillets in a casserole dish. Put some salt and lemon-pepper to taste.

Add the garlic, the onion sliced, the peppers sliced and then put the lemon juice and the olive oil.

Cut tomato to slices and place on top to cover the fish in order not to get burn and remain juicy!

Bake at 350F for 30 minutes approx!

Low Fat Sweet Apple

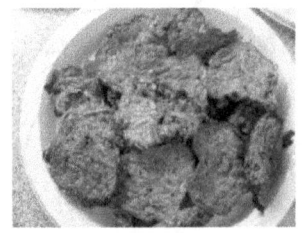

Ingredients
- 3 apples (peeled and shredded)
- 3 -4 tablespoons brown sugar
- 2 large eggs
- 5 -6 tablespoons flour (white or whole)
- 1 tablespoon cinnamon

- cooking spray

Directions

Mix all ingredients.

Spray a baking pan.

Using two tablespoons, form latkes in the pan.

Bake in 350°F.

Turn Latkes over till both sides golden-brown.

Nutrional Values per 1 serving: 59 Calories, 11 grams Carbohydrates, 1.5 grams Protein, 1 grams Fat, 36 Milligrams Cholesterol, 15.25% Fat!

Apple Pie Parfait- Big On Taste, Not Calories!

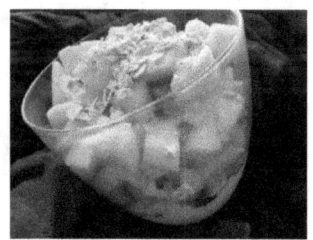

Ingredients
- 1 cup plain low-fat yogurt
- 1 teaspoon honey (approx)
- 1/4 teaspoon apple pie spice

- 1 gala apples, chopped into pieces
- 2 tablespoons rolled oats

Directions

Put the yogurt into the bowl followed by the honey and apple pie spice.

Add the chopped apple and oats, and mix together well.

Serve or refridgerate though I think it's best when the oats are still crunchy.

Simple Sweet Potato Or Pumpkin Muffins (Low Calorie)

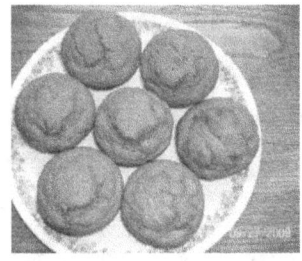

Ingredients
- 1 1/2 cups whole wheat flour
- 1 1/2 teaspoons baking powder
- 3/4 teaspoon baking soda
- 1/3 teaspoon salt
- 1 1/2 teaspoons cinnamon

- 3/4 teaspoon ground ginger
- 1/3 teaspoon nutmeg
- 3/4 cup Egg Beaters egg substitute
- 1 cup sweet potato (mashed)
- 3/4 cup sugar-free maple syrup

Directions

preheat oven to 350.

mix wet ingredients.

mix dry ingredients.

combine wet and dry ingredients until just mixed.

put into lined or greased muffin tin.

bake for 15-20 minutes until toothpick comes out clean.

Jalapeno Rice- Low Fat

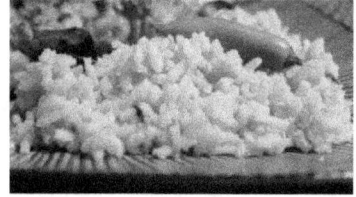

Ingredients
- 1/2 cup brown rice
- 1 cup chicken broth (can or box, homemade or made with bullion)

- 2 jalapeno peppers, chopped. (Remove at least 1/2 the seeds unless you like spicy!)
- 1/2 onion, chopped
- 1/2-1 teaspoon olive oil

Directions

Sautee onion in olive oil.

Combine all ingredients in a pot with a tight-fitting lid, bring to a boil, and then simmer until cooked (30-40 minutes).

ENJOY!

www.ingramcontent.com/pod-product-compliance
Lightning Source LLC
Chambersburg PA
CBHW071442070526
44578CB00001B/190